Introducing Medicines Management

Introducing Medicines Management

Sherri Ogston-Tuck
King's College London

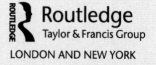
Routledge
Taylor & Francis Group

LONDON AND NEW YORK

First published 2011 by Pearson Education Limited

Published 2013 by Routledge
2 Park Square, Milton Park, Abingdon, Oxon OX14 4RN
711 Third Avenue, New York, NY 10017, USA

Routledge is an imprint of the Taylor & Francis Group, an informa business

ISBN 13: 978-0-273-72088-1 (pbk)

British Library Cataloguing-in-Publication Data
Ogston-Tuck, Sherri.
   Introducing medicines management / Sherri Ogston-Tuck.
      p. cm.
   Includes bibliographical references and index.
   ISBN 978-0-273-72088-1
   1. Drugs–Administration. 2. Nursing. 3. Medical errors–Prevention. I. Title.
   [DNLM: 1. Drug Therapy–nursing. 2. Medication Errors–prevention & control.
   3. Safety Management–methods. WY 100]
   RM125.037 2011
   615'.6–dc22

                                                            2011006093

Library of Congress Cataloging-in-Publication Data

Typeset in 9.5/13.5pt Interstate Light by 35

Contents

Contents

Author's acknowledgements

I would like to acknowledge the students who I have taught over the years and hope this book continues to support others in their learning and nursing practice.

Thank you, Simon, for your support, love and encouragement.

Dedication
For my Father, who always believed in me.

Publisher's acknowledgements

The publishers would like to acknowledge the following organisations for permission to use copyright material:

Chapter 1, p. 7: Nursing and Midwifery Council for 'The code: standards of conduct, performance and ethics for nurses and midwives' (2008).

Chapter 3, Figure 3.1, p. 52: Department of Health for figure 2.4, p. 31 from *Building a Safer NHS for Patients: Improving Medication Safety* (2004), London: The Stationery Office,

Chapter 5, p. 121: *British Journal of Nursing* for 'Central venous access devices: Part 2 For intermediate and long-term use' by K. Scales, *British Journal of Nursing* 19 (5) 2010: S20-5.

Chapter 6
Key sections of the Mental Capacity Act 2010, p. 133, from Mental Capacity Act 2010, www.opsi.gov.uk; main provisions of the Data Protection Act 1998, p. 140, from Data Protection Act 1998, http://www.legislation.gov.uk/ukpga/1998/29/contents. Crown Copyright material is reproduced with permission under the terms of the Click-Use Licence.

Every effort has been made to trace the copyright holders and we apologise in advance for any unintentional omissions. We would be pleased to insert the appropriate acknowledgement in any subsequent edition of this publication.

Preface

Welcome to 'medicines management', which is a relatively new term and is essentially about the issues relating to medicines and health care professionals and patient safety.

Students may not be aware of this term, but it is an integral aspect of nursing and education. The main reason for this is patient safety, which is at the heart of medicines management.

This topic can be linked to many others in the nursing curriculum: professional, ethical and legal issues in health care; health care policy and management; medication administration as a skill; patient care planning and fundamentals of nursing care. You will see from the chapters that this topic is developmental, just as a student is in their journey through their education and training. It is also a good resource for those who have already qualified, and will help to remind health care professionals of their responsibility and safe practice in medicines management.

The goal of this book is to clarify some of the issues in relation to safe steps in medicines management, administration, patient safety and the role of health care professionals in medicines management. It aims to target key issues in patient safety and help you to understand how mistakes can happen and how they can be avoided. *Introducing Medicines Management* contains six chapters that are relatively short and interactive to help you engage with the topic and participate in activities to test your knowledge and help in your learning along the way. This book starts with an introduction to the role of the nurse in **Chapter 1**. Understanding the role of the nurse and our 'professional' capacity is vitally important. Clearly, the professional role will develop and change as you progress in your studies and move from 'student nurse' to 'qualified nurse'. Professional limitations will be discussed and new terms, such as accountability, duty of care, and negligence, introduced. Further, an overview of the law and pertinent legislation will be necessary, such that professional and legal duty of care is made clear and understood. This chapter will help you to focus on your professional development. It is therefore vital that you understand your professional limitations, the law, and how medicines management is shaped by our role and responsibility to ensure safe practice and a high standard of care. This chapter will introduce you to the Nursing and Midwifery Council and explain the role and purpose of this professional regulating body. It will examine some of the related legal, professional and ethical issues. This will help you to engage in and explore the nurse's role and responsibilities in medicines management.

Chapter 2 takes the nurse on a journey that explores how we 'fit' within the health care profession and how the inter-professional team is a network of support, each thread a vital link in care delivery. Teamwork is an important element and essential if we are to provide safe and effective care. Therefore how we work together, how we communicate and manage medicines, is a responsibility of everyone in health care. This chapter will invite you to consider other roles and limitations and participate in activities in order to engage and challenge you.

Chapter 3 looks at systems. A safe systems approach is central to safe practice, and within medicines management it is a key issue for discussion. This will be explored and safe systems discussed, which will include a discussion and interactive activity on 'The Five Rights' and help you to reflect on other steps that are essential for safe practice in medicines management.

Chapter 4 will then identify errors that are a result of poor practice, unsafe practice or are a result of systems that fail. This is an important chapter, with the intention to decrease error incidence by increasing awareness. Interactive activities will help you identify types of error, the cause of error and their incidence. In this chapter, it will be important to gain insight into how mistakes can happen and, more importantly, how they can be prevented in the first instance. Often it is only when something goes wrong that we realise a mistake has occurred; the consequence of this is unfortunate because it is often too late to prevent harm or injury to the patient. However, awareness and learning from mistakes can prevent their recurrence. This chapter will include tips for safe practice and practical steps to problem solving and medicine calculations.

Chapter 5 addresses key issues that target pharmacological principles. This is a vital element of nursing, where our duty of care is not to harm the patient, and our professional role requires us to promote health and prevent illness. Therefore issues surrounding patient education will be addressed. Further, you will need to have an understanding of key pharmacological principles and key terms such as pharmacotherapeutics, pharmacodynamics and pharmacokinetics. Interactive activities will help you to explore your current role, as a student in patient education and health promotion, which is a continuum in nursing and in your career. This chapter will also cover aspects of medicines management and routes of medicine administration. This will complement the pharmacological principles addressed in this chapter.

Chapter 6 is the final chapter, to consolidate what you have learned and to consider how this information will take you forward and prepare you for qualification. It is essential that nurses are confident in their clinical decision making and communication skills. Our professional role and duty of care requires that we advocate for patients in our care and that we ensure safe and effective standards of practice and care. Thus, this chapter will help you to reflect on your role and how it has and will change. It will focus on effective communication skills, which are vital particularly in challenging situations. Some tips and practical components will make up the activities and help in your learning and personal reflection.

Introduction

Medication management encompasses the interrelated elements of managing and administering medicines and the intricacies in the provision of safe and effective patient care. Medicines are fundamental to the management and prevention of disease, therapeutic treatment and intervention for illness. Their management is therefore an essential component of care, underpinning safety. Medicines management is the responsibility of all health care professionals.

The Medicines and Healthcare Products Regulatory Agency (MHRA 2004) defines medicines management as the clinical, cost-effective and safe use of medicines to ensure patients get the maximum benefit from the medicines they need, while at the same time minimising patient harm. Thus, management involves organisation, supervision and administration, from a collaborative and effective inter-professional team.

This book aims to explore medicines management and to give nurses a greater understanding of their professional role and responsibilities. In doing this it will provide awareness of and underpinning for the knowledge required to understand the complexities and challenges of medicines management and factors essential to safe practice and effective care delivery.

The role of the nurse is expanding and changing, as are our communities and the world we live in. This brings with it greater challenges for health care professionals and undoubtedly this will have a direct impact on patients and their care.

Key learning outcomes:

- To enable practitioners to develop their knowledge of the nursing role and the extent of this in relation to professional accountability and responsibilities in medicines management.

- To provide practitioners with the confidence to explore the safe process of medicines management and apply integral steps, so that nurses and the health care team see this as a fluid concept.

1

- To provide greater awareness of the interrelationship between the patient, the medicine and the prescription as a fundamental systems approach, in order to understand how this relates to effective medicines management.

- To raise an awareness of the importance of recognising the potential for errors and to encourage effective use of mechanisms of reporting to identify and learn from clinical incidents and preventative measures.

- To reflect on the challenges that health care professionals face today, gain knowledge and skills for effective communication, and improve teamwork and leadership, all of which are integral to safe medicines management, delivery and patient care.

References

MHRA (2004) *Medicines for Human Use (Clinical Trials) Regulations 2004*, Medicines and Healthcare Products Regulatory Agency (www.mhra.gov.uk)

Chapter 1

The professional role of the nurse

When you have completed this chapter you should:

- understand what is meant by 'professional role'
- understand the meaning of accountability, responsibility and duty of care
- have an awareness of your role, including expectations and limitations
- have an understanding of legal and professional principles
- have an awareness of legal, ethical and professional issues in medicines management

Your starting point

Answer the following and begin reflecting on what it is to be a nurse.

1. What are three characteristics you possess that are important to being a nurse?

   ....

   ....

2. What does 'professional' mean to you?

   ....

   ....

3. Define 'responsible'.

   ....

   ....

4. What is it to be accountable?

   ....

   ....

5. Do you think responsibility and accountability are different?

   Yes ☐   No ☐   Unsure ☐

6. Think of a limitation you have now, in your current year of study as a student nurse or in your role as a nurse.

   ....

7. What are three expectations the patient has of the nurse caring for them?

   ....

   ....

   ....

8. Are nurses legally accountable?

   Yes ☐   No ☐   Unsure ☐

Introduction

Welcome to medicines management – a term that is often misunderstood and unclear, but which has a powerful impact on nursing and the health care profession.

Let us start by trying to understand what nursing is. It is the promotion of health and well-being, which, although a useful phrase, throws up a lot of questions and ethical issues for nurses and health care professionals. Our duty as nurses is not to harm our patients. Patients in our care trust us with their health and well-being. Therefore, nurses undertake an enormous responsibility in caring for people and protecting them from harm and helping them to get better. But is that all we do? This highlights the importance of belonging to a 'profession'.

Professional practice

The key terms 'professional accountability' and 'professional behaviour' stem from the standards of care that encompass 'professionalism'. So, a good starting point to understanding what it is that nurses do and what they are is to consider how one respects others and their autonomy.

ACTIVITY 1.1

If you were a patient (or have been) how would you want to be treated by health care professionals?

....

....

Do you have an expectation of the treatment and care you will receive?

....

....

What is important in regard to 'your autonomy'?

....

....

This raises moral, legal and ethical dilemmas and makes up fundamental aspects of the professional dimension. By reflecting on what and how nurses relate to their patients/clients, and indeed the public, gives rise to one's professionalism and indeed one's accountability.

Being a professional is therefore about the way in which we act, as it relates to issues of morality, ethics and law. Professions establish themselves through regulation and formal legislation, as a means of protection for the public and to ensure safe standards of care. Therefore, being professional is about being proficient, skilled, trained and practised. It allows one to be specialised or considered an expert in something. It is about being licensed or certified. It is a status; one of high regard wherein professional practice is recognised, maintained, monitored and safeguarded.

The Nursing and Midwifery Council

For nurses, this professional status requires registration with the Nursing and Midwifery Council (NMC), whose purpose is to ensure that registrants have met the requirements and standards set by the Council through education and training. It means that the registrants can demonstrate and maintain these standards in their practice.

ACTIVITY 1.2

Access the NMC website at www.nmc-uk.org. Search the site to identify what the NMC is, its function and its purpose.

The NMC Code is the foundation of good nursing and midwifery practice, and a key tool in safeguarding the health and well-being of the public (NMC, 2008a). This would have come up in your search and it is a vital document providing guidance and standards that nurses must adhere to and demonstrate in their patient care. Protecting the public is of the highest importance and, as a result, nurses must demonstrate safe and effective care at all times.

The Council's main function is to set standards for practice and provide professional guidance, in order to protect the public. The Code is about being professional, about being accountable, and about being able to justify your decisions (NMC, 2008a).

The very nature of what we do as nurses demands that we are practising in a way that is safe and professional. The registry is open to public scrutiny, wherein members of the public are freely able to access information about registrants. This includes practice standards, fitness for practice, adherence to professional guidelines and professional conduct. The NMC is integral to setting fitness-for-practice standards for registrants and ensuring these standards are met.

'The people in your care must be able to trust you with their health and wellbeing.

To justify that trust, you must

- *make the care of people your first concern, treating them as individuals and respecting their dignity*
- *work with others to protect and promote the health and wellbeing of those in your care, their families and carers, and the wider community*
- *provide a high standard of practice and care at all times*
- *be open and honest, act with integrity and uphold the reputation of your profession'*

(NMC, 2008a)

As a professional, you are personally accountable for actions and omissions in your practice and you must always be able to justify your decisions. You must always act lawfully, whether those laws relate to your professional practice or to your personal life. Failure to comply with this Code may bring your fitness to practise into question and endanger your registration.

ACTIVITY 1.3

From the bullet points in the extract above, give an example of how you would demonstrate this in clinical practice.

....

....

....

....

....

....

Professional accountability

The very fact that as registrants to the NMC we belong to a professional body links our practice to conduct which could be described not only as safe but also as legal. In addition, legislation provides legal parameters and standards of practice that nurses must abide by. Our practice is measured against these standards, which is why nurses are held to account, are liable, and are scrutinised by the public and the profession. Importantly, then, the level of professional responsibility is directly related to the role of the practitioner and their area of clinical expertise. Clearly, the greater the practitioner's responsibility, that is, the more expert and/or specialised their practice, then the greater the scrutiny to which they will be subject and accountability to which they will be held.

It is therefore essential that one understands what is meant by being responsible, and likewise what is meant by accountability and liability.

- **Accountability** can be defined as being responsible for something or to someone (NMC, 2008a). It is an obligation to give reckoning or explanation for one's actions.
- **Responsibility** can be defined as a legal or moral obligation to take care of something or to carry out a duty; liable to be blamed for loss or failure.

Professional roles and professional duty of care encompass professional accountability. Nurses are accountable for what they do and for what they do not do and are personally accountable for their own practice.

ACTIVITY 1.4

On the diagram below indicate in each circle who you think the nurse is accountable to.

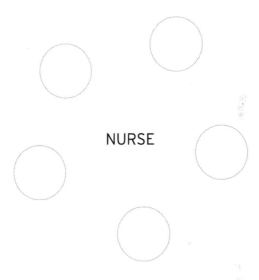

NURSE

Professional accountability is inescapable in that it requires an individual to justify their actions and omissions. An omission of appropriate care could be seen as being as serious as the provision of inappropriate care. Culpability is often associated with being responsible or liable, but it also means guilty or in the wrong or to blame.

Can a nurse be accountable, responsible and culpable all at the same time?

Yes ☐   No ☐

The four main arenas of professional accountability are:

1. To the patient

2. To the public

3. To the profession

4. To the employer.

These arenas are linked to areas in law - employment law, civil law and criminal law.

You are also accountable to yourself and to the professional registering body for nurses and midwives, the NMC.

In some practice areas, such as nurse-led clinics or where nurses manage a team or prescribe, the nurses are taking on more responsibility and therefore have greater accountability.

ACTIVITY 1.5

Consider your mentor while you are a student in practice. Do you think she/he has a level of accountability for you and your actions/omissions?

....

....

What is your responsibility as a student nurse? Do you think this is shared with your mentor?

....

....

It is important, therefore, that nurses are aware of their responsibilities and their level of accountability, how this changes and the impact it has, particularly where something could go wrong.

Self-regulation is the legal framework for the nursing profession and is the current regulatory system for all nurses and midwives. It is therefore a requirement that all practising nurses and midwives be on the registry of the NMC and maintain a professional registration with the Council.

Why is registration with the NMC necessary?

It is this professional registering body which maintains and sets the standards of care and fitness for practice of those registered and it does this to ensure that the delivery and provision of patient care is safe, effective and competent. Registrants are duty-bound by the NMC standards and must demonstrate professional practice at all times.

ACTIVITY 1.6

Review the legal framework for nurses and midwives and the Parliamentary Acts, identifying the most relevant legislation that has led to the NMC regulating body.

....

....

....

....

....

....

When things go wrong

The protection of the public is paramount, and the NMC has a key role in monitoring the standards of patient care and maintaining the standards of the registrants. Often it is not until something goes wrong that one thinks of the law, or of the effect that the incident will have on their registration.

ACTIVITY 1.7

Do you have your driving licence? ....

If yes, how long have you had it and ask yourself, do you drive in the same way now as when you were taught?

....

....

If you answered no, ask yourself why not?

....

....

Would you describe your driving as careless? Or reckless?

....

....

Now let's add to this theme. What do you think it means to be careless or reckless as a nurse? Is this the result of taking 'shortcuts'?

Do you think this is the same as being negligent?

Yes ☐   No ☐

Negligence can be described as any act of carelessness, lack of regard or lack of insight which can lead to patient harm. It is the degree of patient harm that determines the significance of the negligent act. This is important, because negligence describes a particular type of fault. This can be either criminal, leading to criminal prosecution, or civil, leading to an action in the civil courts for compensation and damages.

In nursing practice, however, it is rare that an act of carelessness or lack of regard would result in criminal proceedings and there are very few cases where nurses have been prosecuted in a criminal court. Most cases concern the civil law of negligence (law of tort).

 ACTIVITY 1.8

Can you recall a case of a nurse, reported in the media, who was prosecuted in a criminal court of law or in a civil court of law? Let's review the case of Beverly Allitt.

Ms Allitt was convicted of murdering four children, of attempting to murder three others and of causing grievous bodily harm to six more. She was sentenced to life imprisonment on every count (Clothier Report, 1994).

This is an example of how all arenas of accountability can be exercised: Allitt was removed from the NMC register, relieved of her duties without pay by her employer and was prosecuted for murder in a criminal court of law, and the families of those who suffered harm were compensated in clinical negligence claims.

How does this make you feel regarding this nurse, her actions and the profession of which you are (will be) a part?

....

....

....

....

....

....

Key differences between criminal and civil cases and the legal elements that need to be satisfied for each:

- *Criminal law* – This requires two elements: the act and the intent. Often these cases involve serious crimes such as murder or manslaughter and other criminal offences such as grievous bodily harm, assault and battery. Criminal law proceedings require proof 'beyond reasonable doubt'.
- *Clinical negligence claims* – It is the elements of the tort of negligence that must be satisfied where the claimant must show that the defendant owed a duty of care; that they breached that duty of care; and that the breach caused some injury, loss or damage. Civil proceedings are based on 'reasonableness' and a 'balance of probabilities'.

The incidence of litigation by patients and families seeking damages for clinical negligence and loss is on the rise. The law functions to protect the public from wrongdoing, so when a patient is harmed or injured, that person may seek compensation for the wrongdoing. Often this is the result of adverse incidents, error in practice or acts of negligence, where the similarity of the outcome for any of these untoward events is patient harm.

Let's put these elements into perspective:

1. Duty of care established.
2. Breach of that duty of care.
3. Patient harm.

Duty of care established

In the clinical area, it is important to ascertain one's accountability first and foremost and, as such, one's duty of care is therefore established. The general principles for breach of duty for a professional can be applied from the Bolam Principle (Dimond, 2008): the ubiquitous test. This is not only a rule of substantive law, such that it defines what amounts to adequate care, but it is also about evidence and indicates how the courts will determine whether adequate care has been given or not.

Breach of that duty of care

Let us consider an instance where a nurse is the delegated and named nurse to specific patients on the ward or unit. The named nurse is designated, for instance, to the 'red team'. Therefore this nurse would have a duty of care to the six patients on this named team. Depending on the nurse's level of knowledge, expertise and experience, their responsibility may vary, but once they accept responsibility, they have an established duty of care. If this nurse should then leave the ward without informing another nurse, or fail to report a change in a patient's condition or fail to give the medications to one of those patients as prescribed, then a breach in that duty of care to that patient on that named team would arise.

Patient harm

Establishing patient harm is less complicated; it is, however, the degree of harm suffered that will determine the consequences and outcome. Failing to report a change in the patient's condition may be seen as insignificant or be overlooked; however if this is a vital statistic that leads to cardiac arrest and death, the implications for the nurse, professionally and legally, are manifold. A preventable accident, such as a patient fall, caused by the failure of the nurse to inform another that they are leaving the ward, could result in a simple bruise or minor concussion. However, if the fall led to a broken limb or major complication and a prolonged patient stay, or indeed if it compromised the patient's health and well-being, then the implications of the nurse's negligence become significant. Similarly, missing medications may be an oversight and are often not reported, but the omission could have devastating consequences for the patient, for example if the medication is to maintain a therapeutic heart rate or blood pressure, or to treat a fever or infection.

Clinical negligence claims are a financial burden on the NHS and cause a loss in patient confidence. It is therefore essential that nurses are acutely aware of their professional accountability, and their limitations.

ACTIVITY 1.9

Access the NMC website at www.nmc-uk.org. Review the outcomes of misconduct cases and annual reports for those registrants who are no longer on the registry, suspended or undergoing professional misconduct hearings and fitness-for-practice hearings.

ACTIVITY 1.10

Read the scenario below and consider the questions based on what you have read so far.

A patient is administered 40 times the prescribed amount of an opioid analgesic by a nurse who has been practising on a surgical ward for five years. The nurse has not attended a recent update in medicines management and failed to calculate the correct dose or check this with another nurse before administering the drug. The patient suffered cardiac arrest and was transferred to the intensive care unit.

Apply the principles of tort. Do you think the nurse is negligent?

What do you think would be the consequences for this nurse as a result of this?

....

....

....

....

....

....

Understanding your limitations

It is important that practitioners are aware of their limitations, and these are largely reflected in their role. It is true that the role of the nurse is expanding, but within that role the individual must be aware of their professional boundaries and restrictions. For example, a junior or newly qualified nurse would have limitations that prevent them from accepting greater responsibility, such as taking charge of the team and all of the patients on a ward.

A senior nurse or ward manager will have limitations too. For example, a ward manager would not necessarily be permitted to prescribe medication or to insert a central line, but they may direct others in a cardiac arrest and take the lead on the management of the patient in this event.

Understanding one's professional boundaries and limitations is paramount. These restrictions may be varied and largely dictated by one's job description or contract of employment. It is important to understand and work within these at all times.

There may also be times when the role of the nurse requires delegation of tasks to others or indeed taking orders from someone else. Again, understanding one's limitations is important, and often this limits what one can and cannot do, even under the instruction of another. Of course this may change somewhat in an emergency situation, and delegation is aided by algorithms and approved interventions, such as in resuscitation. The nurse acting on another's instructions must accept responsibility, and indeed accountability, for their actions.

Making ethical decisions

At the beginning of this chapter you were asked to consider autonomy. Respecting patient autonomy is one of the four key ethical principles in decision making. This is of particular relevance when faced with difficult decisions that are not straightforward and may present challenges to us that force us to reflect on our own moral and ethical paradigm.

There are four ethical principles that can help in decision making:

1. autonomy

2. beneficence

3. non-maleficence

4. justice.

These constitute a utilitarian principalist approach to decision making where ethical and moral paradigms conflict with the professional and legal dimension. The principle of respect for autonomy entails taking into account and giving consideration to the patient's views on their treatment. However, this is not an all or nothing concept. The difficulty lies in our understanding as professionals that some treatment may involve some harm, even if minimal, but the harm should not be disproportionate to the benefits of the proposed treatment.

Perhaps what we need to do is ask ourselves, would the patient be harmed by the treatment, and does the benefit of the treatment outweigh the risks and costs to the patient? Respect for autonomy can at times clash with the other principles, particularly when the patient makes a decision that the health care professional does not think will benefit the patient or is not in the patient's best interests.

From a legal point of view, the wishes of a competent patient cannot be overridden in their best interests. But how do we feel about, for example, forcibly restraining a patient in order to administer their medicine? If the patient does not comply with the treatment, would it be impractical to carry it out? To what harm would the patient come without the treatment? Is the treatment in their best interests? Unfortunately, there are no straightforward answers. But we can prepare ourselves better by trying three simple steps:

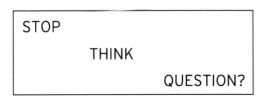

These are three simple steps where stopping and thinking about the situation, and questioning can influence how we make decisions that involve our patients. Understanding ethics helps health care professionals decide *how* to act; how they ought to respect autonomy, avoid harming, where possible benefit, and to consider (fairly) the interests of those affected.

ACTIVITY 1.11

Below are the four principles listed, with a brief explanation for each one. From what you have read so far, try to match these up correctly by placing a number against the corresponding letter.

A. Autonomy   ....

B. Beneficence   ....

C. Non-maleficence   ....

D. Justice   ....

1. Distributing benefits, risks and costs fairly; the notion that patients in similar positions should be treated in a similar manner.

2. Avoiding the causation of harm; the health care professional should not harm the patient.

3. Respecting the decision-making capacities of autonomous persons; enabling individuals to make reasoned informed choices.

4. Balancing of benefits; the health care professional should act to benefit their patient.

Chapter summary

This chapter has focused on you and what you will become or already are: a nurse, a health care professional. It has clarified what constitutes 'professional' and the importance and relevance of this in relation to safeguarding patients. This chapter has identified important terms that apply to your professional duty of care and issues surrounding safe, effective and lawful patient care. When nurses fail to meet standards of care, our professional registering body (the NMC) and indeed higher elements of the law may challenge our conduct and performance. Sometimes it helps to reflect on our role, boundaries and limitations. Sometimes it helps to apply principles to help in our decision making when we are providing patient care.

Medicines management encompasses these principles: not to harm; to give medicines that benefit the patient, and to do so safely and conscientiously. When you are about to administer a medicine to a patient, stop and think. Think about the patient and think about the drug. The drug could potentially cause harm or lead to some discomfort for the patient, but it also has some benefit for the patient that may outweigh the risks. The patient trusts us, with their health and well-being (NMC, 2008a).

Therefore our duty of care is not to harm our patients. Decision making needs to be considerate of the patient and decisions should be made in their best interests wherever possible. This embodies the characteristics of professionalism, it reminds us of our responsibility and accountability, and it is at the heart of safe and effective patient care.

So what have you learned?

Let's do a quick check. Here are five short questions – just tick whether each of these statements is true or false.

1. The NMC is a responsible body of people that protects nurses when things go wrong.

   True ☐   False ☐

2. Acting in a way that is shown to be careless or reckless and which results in patient harm can be described as negligent and may lead to further investigation, litigation and jeopardise your nursing registration.

   True ☐   False ☐

3. Nurses are accountable to the public, to their patients, to their professional registering body and to their employer.

   True ☐   False ☐

4. Civil law cases must satisfy three elements based on a balance of probabilities whereas criminal law cases must prove the elements of the crime beyond reasonable doubt.

   True ☐   False ☐

5. The four principles of ethical decision making are: respect for autonomy; beneficence; non-maleficence; justice.

   True ☐   False ☐

References and key texts

Beauchamp, T.L. and Childress, J.F. (2009) *Principles of Biomedical Ethics*, 6th edn. Oxford: Oxford University Press.

Clothier Report (1994) *The Allitt Inquiry: Independent inquiry relating to death and injury on the children's ward at Grantham and Kesteven General Hospital during the period February to April 1991*. London: HMSO.

Dimond, B. (ed.) (2008) *Legal Aspects of Nursing*, 5th edn. London: Pearson.

NMC (Nursing and Midwifery Council) (2008a) *The Code: Standards of Conduct, Performance and Ethics for Nurses and Midwives*. London: NMC.

NMC (Nursing and Midwifery Council) (2008b) *Standards for Medicines Management*. London: NMC.

Tingle, J. and Cribb, A. (2007) *Nursing Law and Ethics*. Oxford: Blackwell.

Additional reading

Boylan-Kemp, J. (2009) 'The legal system. Part 2: It's not just for lawyers'. *British Journal of Nursing* 18 (3): 178-80.

Department of Health (1991) *The Patient's Charter*. London: The Stationery Office.

Department of Health (1991) *Saving Lives: Our Healthier Nation*. London: The Stationery Office.

Department of Health (1999) *Making a Difference: Strengthening the Nursing, Midwifery and Health Contribution to Health and Healthcare*. London: The Stationery Office.

Griffith, R. and Tengnah, C. (2010) *Law and Professional Issues in Nursing*, 2nd edn. Exeter: Learning Matters.

Griffith, R., Griffith, H. and Jordan, S. (2003) 'Administration of medicines. Part 1: The law and nursing'. *Nursing Standard* 16: 47-53.

McHale, J. and Tingle, J. (2007) *Law and Nursing*, 3rd edn. Edinburgh: Elsevier.

NMC (Nursing and Midwifery Council) (2004) *Advice Sheet: Medicines Management*. London: NMC.

Savage, J. and Moore, L. (2004) *Interpreting Accountability: An Ethnographic Study of Practice Nurses, Accountability and Multidisciplinary Team Decision-Making in the Context of Clinical Governance*. London: RCN.

Thompson, I.E., Melia, K.M. and Boyd, K.M. (2001) *Nursing Ethics*, 4th edn. Oxford: Churchill Livingstone.

Wheat, K. (2009) 'Applying ethical principles in healthcare practice'. *British Journal of Nursing* 18 (17): 1062-3.

Websites

http://www.dh.gov.uk

http://www.mhra.gov.uk

http://www.nhsla.com

http://www.nmc-uk.org

http://www.opsi.gov.uk

Chapter 2

The inter-professional team

When you have completed this chapter you should:

- understand what makes up the inter-professional role and responsibilities
- understand professional boundaries
- understand the meaning of teamwork and how this is fundamental to health care delivery
- have an understanding of effective communication

Your starting point

Answer the following and begin reflecting on 'teamwork' and 'effective communication'.

1. Write down a definition of 'teamwork'.

   ....

   ....

2. What does the Code (NMC, 2008) state in relation to teamwork and professional standards of care?

   ....

   ....

3. Reflect on your experiences in clinical practice. Can you give three examples of poor teamwork?

   ....

   ....

   ....

4. What could you do to improve teamwork?

   ....

   ....

   ....

   ....

5. Identify at least six members of an 'inter-professional team'.

   ....

   ....

   ....

   ....

6. What do you think your role is within the inter-professional team?

....

....

....

7. Do you think everyone on the team has the same professional goal?

Yes ☐   No ☐   Unsure ☐

If yes, then explain what it is.

....

....

....

....

....

Introduction

The inter-professional team is a good starting point for this chapter because it is where we 'fit' into health care but it is also where 'team' becomes an essential ingredient to efficient and effective health care delivery. Recall that in Chapter 1, we defined medicines management which identifies that essentially everyone has a responsibility for the safe, effective use and management of medicines.

This means that everyone who is involved in the delivery of health care bears this responsibility. The nurse is a core component in the delivery of health care, and an essential member of the interprofessional team. The other members will be identified and discussed in this chapter, as will the concept of teamwork. Bear in mind that this discussion should encompass safety and will therefore prepare you for the next chapter as well as develop the knowledge and understanding you gained from the previous chapter.

Who's who in the inter-professional team

Let's start with your answer for question 5 above, where you were asked to provide at least six identified members of the inter-professional team. The two most popular answers would include doctors and nurses. But who else makes up the team and why are they important?

Let us review 'who's who'.

Pharmacists

The role of prescribing was in the past fulfilled by doctors; however, a range of health care workers can now prescribe independently from the British National Formulary (BNF). Pharmacists can also prescribe as a supplementary prescriber.

The pharmacist is an essential resource to any ward or clinical environment and within the community health care setting. Pharmacists possess sound knowledge of medicines and their use. They are integral to patient education and safe systems of dispensing medicines, and are largely associated with drug formulations, drug preparation and managing adverse incidents and errors. They are an essential element in the safe delivery of medicines.

Pharmacists have a unique role as a key checking point in safe systems: when reviewing prescriptions, preparing medicines for use such as nutritional feeds and other routes of medicine use, antibiotic therapy, anticoagulants, pain management and insulin therapy, and any other medications patients will require.

Their wealth of knowledge and expertise can support other members of the inter-professional team and indeed the patient in regard to the prescription, medication regimen, drug interactions, preparation and contra-indications, side effects and indeed adverse events. They have also developed in their role as non-medical prescribers. Pharmacists and technicians abide by a professional code of ethics from the Royal Pharmaceutical Society that ensures patient safety, safe decision making and collaborative working (RPSGB, 2007). Chief pharmacists and pharmaceutical advisers have key leadership roles, but making medication practice safer needs engagement by doctors, nurses and other staff, as well as the pharmacy team.

Key roles of the pharmacist in medicines management:

- Review patient information and prescribed medication
- Check prescription
    - Drug name
    - Dose
    - Route
    - Frequency / valid period
    - Additional comments
- Dispense prescribed medication
    - Review and monitor drug regimen
    - Patient education (medicines on discharge)
    - Inter-professional education
    - Adverse incidents

Doctors

Doctors have a clearly defined role in medicines management and are the key prescribers for all medications, treatments and interventions in patient care. Doctors are registered with the General Medical Council (GMC) and must adhere to that body's code of conduct (GMC, 2010). The GMC's statutory purpose is to protect, promote and maintain the health and safety of the public by ensuring proper standards in the practice of medicine (GMC, 2010).

Key roles of the doctor in medicines management:

- Obtain comprehensive history from the patient
    - Medical history
    - Medication history
- Pharmacological management of care
- Treatment and interventions
    - Prescribe medications
    - Monitor medications and their effect
    - Review medication regimen

Who else?

There are numerous health care and non-health-care professionals who work as part of a team within health care delivery: physiotherapists;

various technicians; phlebotomists; occupational therapists; nutritionists; health care assistants; porters; surgeons; anaesthetists; psychiatrists; ambulance attendants; radiologists; paramedics; specialist teams in pain, patient falls, stroke, diabetes; language therapists; various managers and educationalists; consultants; junior and senior practitioners; students of all disciplines; auxiliary staff and community care workers. The list could go on.

Each and every one of these individuals has a link with medicines management although they may not have a direct responsibility to the patient and their care. Exposure to medicines; infusions of fluids, drugs or blood products; enteral feedings and nutrition; syringes including those in use or discarded, or left at the patient bedside – all equate to responsibility to ensure potential errors are minimised and reported. Each has a responsibility to actively minimise risk from medicines found, discarded, left at the bedside or not in use.

The importance of teamwork

Before we discuss the role of the nurse, let us review why the team is fundamental to our health care and delivery of care and, indeed, to the patient. Patients present to the NHS in a variety of shapes, age, sizes, hereditary background, cultures, ethnicity, illness, diseases, ailment, injury, conditions, and so on. The human condition is complex, as is modern medicine. Together then, we strive to treat, cure, help, manage, prevent illness, promote health, educate, intervene, operate, investigate, medicate, cure or alleviate the presenting problem(s). It requires a multitude of skill, expertise, knowledge and experience. This is reflected in the inter-professional team and their provision of health care service to patients.

What makes a team effective?

Other words to describe 'effective' include useful, valuable, efficient, successful. In health care, teamwork has been defined as a dynamic process involving two or more health care professionals with complementary backgrounds and skills, sharing common health goals and exercising concerted physical and mental effort in assessing, planning or evaluating patient care.

The NMC indicates that nurses must work effectively as part of a team (NMC, 2008). In doing this, they must work cooperatively within teams and respect the skills, expertise and contributions of colleagues; share skills and experience for the benefit of their colleagues; consult and take advice from colleagues when appropriate; treat colleagues fairly and without discrimination; and make referrals to other health care practitioners in the best interests of patients in their care.

Teamwork requires key components in order for it to effective such as good communication; coordination; balance of contribution and expertise; mutual support; effort; and cohesion. In order to be meaningful, communication requires key participants – a sender and a receiver – and it requires a message. It is not only verbal communication that constitutes effective communication but also the ability to pick up on non-verbal cues, body language and eye contact. In health care it is vital that people working together with a common goal are clear in their communication and that this includes the patient whenever and wherever possible.

In medicine administration, engaging with the patient can help to minimise risk, clarify care needs and prove beneficial to the overall outcome of patient care. Teams need to be inclusive of the patient, their family and carer(s). How we work together and coordinate patient care is equally necessary. Just think of the roles and responsibilities of the inter-professional team and how this comes together in medication management. Example 2.1 below will help to illustrate this.

Further, it is vital that an effective team should not only work together but also support each other. In medicines management there is a great deal to understand and to know with regard to patient treatment and care and indeed their medicines. Drawing on others' knowledge and expertise can improve decision making and collaboration that is in the patient's best interests. A cohesive team may appear effortless in their ability to work alongside each other, minimising risks to patients and managing their medicines effectively and safely.

A team can, however, break down, change, falter and fragment. It is then no longer effective and functioning as it should.

What do you think might contribute to the breakdown of a team?

What might be the consequence of this?

In Chapter 1, we discussed accountability and responsibility and the outcomes when things go wrong. Often it is the person on the receiving end of our care, treatment, intervention, etc. that suffers harm, injury, neglect, a misdiagnosis or worse, death. Medicines management is everyone's responsibility and it is important to remember that a good team is effective where teamwork can make a difference and improve the outcomes for the patient. Example 2.1 provides a simple example of how this works.

Example 2.1

The doctor sees the patient, gathers a medical history, orders some tests and investigations to confirm a diagnoses. The patient is then admitted to the ward and is prescribed medicines and various treatments.

The pharmacist reviews the patient's prescription, sees the patient and confirms the medication history, and verifies medication and dosages prescribed. Additional comments are made to the prescription regarding one or two familiar drugs the patient is on regularly and adds instructions with another medication in relation to taking this on an empty stomach.

The nurse greets the patient, ensures he is settled into his new surroundings and is comfortable. The nurse completes an admission history and takes observation data, explains routines to the patient and confirms the patient's identity with the prescription card.

The nurse reviews the prescription, having established that she/he is familiar with the patient history and the prescribed medicines for this patient. The nurse acknowledges key steps to ensure this is the correct patient, the correct medications for this time, the correct drug name, dose and route, and confirms that the patient has not eaten or taken the medicines already and verifies that the patient is familiar with the medicines prescribed.

The patient takes his medicines having been informed of possible side effects, medication use and outcomes, benefits and risks. The nurse documents that the patient has taken the medicine prescribed.

The nurse returns 40 minutes later to check on the patient and notices a slight rash has appeared.

The nurse informs the pharmacist that the patient developed a slight rash from what may be the new antibiotic prescribed. The doctor is duly informed and the patient is prescribed an antihistamine. The nurse asks the student nurse to check the patient's observations and monitor his oxygen levels and to report anything unusual. The pharmacist reviews the prescription. The physiotherapist who is seeing another patient is informed by the patient's family that he has never had antibiotics before; other than penicillin, but it was a long time ago. They did recall the patient suffering from a red rash and indicated he hadn't taken it again since. The physiotherapist reports this to the nurse. The nurse documents this and informs the pharmacist and the doctor. The antibiotic is discontinued and the doctor and pharmacist consult as to another course of treatment and await blood results taken by the phlebotomist.

ACTIVITY 2.1

Read Example 2.1. Does this reflect teamwork? Why?

....

....

....

....

....

....

Role of the nurse

The nurse is at the very centre of patient care and has a vital role in the safe delivery and effectiveness of patient care. Nurses and midwives are regulated by the Nursing and Midwifery Council (NMC), setting standards for practice, education and registration for nurses and midwives in England, Wales, Scotland, Northern Ireland and the Islands (NMC, 2010).

Although the role of the nurse was once limited and to a large degree under the direction and orders of a doctor, it has since developed in professional integrity and has expanded significantly. In medicines management, nurses are primarily responsible for administering the prescribed medicines. However, today we can see how this task has also developed. It now encompasses:

- Non-medical prescribing of medicines – since May 2006, over 30,000 nurses have been prescribing medicines (NMC, 2010)
- Clinical decision making in pain management and dosage or drug formulation adjustments
- Dosage monitoring in coagulation and diabetic therapy and dosage adjustments
- Critical clinical decision making in resuscitation and life-saving treatments
- Interpreting clinical measurements for drug therapy, inotropic titration and other infusion therapies.

Can you think of any other examples of how the nurse's role has developed within medicines management?

ACTIVITY 2.2

Reflect on your role and the extent to which you are involved in medicines management and your responsibilities. Jot down your thoughts.

....

....

....

....

....

....

It should be clear that the nurse plays a vital role in medicine administration. This begins with the patient first and foremost, and the patient-nurse relationship is established and develops between nurses and their patients. Patients put a great deal of trust into the nurse and it is important that the nurse maintains that trust, demonstrates professional behaviour, respects the patient and ensures their dignity, trust and confidentiality is upheld.

Nurses are at the forefront of the initial patient meeting and are largely responsible in the initiation and instigation of the patient journey in developing the patient care plan/pathway; providing treatment and interventions; monitoring, assessing and evaluating patients and their response to our care and treatment.

Key responsibilities of the nurse in medicines management:

- Review patient history and patient care plan

- Review the prescription chart
  - The prescription chart should be clearly written, legible and unambiguous
  - Verify the identity of the patient and any allergies
  - Understand the indication and therapeutic effect of the drug(s) prescribed; verify that it is the correct dose, route and time

- Patient education
  - Confirm the patients knowledge and understanding of the medicine to be given
  - Obtain consent

- Administer medications prescribed
  - Prepare medication to be given using a non-touch technique having washed hands or having donned non-sterile gloves if indicated
  - Ensure equipment is prepared and appropriate
  - Understand how to use the equipment
  - Check expiry dates on all associated equipment: additives, syringes, etc.
  - Dispose of equipment according to safe handling procedures
  - Wash your hands

- Monitor the patient's response
  - Understand variables and parameters for which the drug may have an effect, such as change in heart rate or blood pressure, etc.
  - Assess the patient and the effect of the drug
  - Monitor the patient for any side effects or adverse effects of the drug administered
- Document
  - The nurse must witness and confirm the patient has taken the medicine before updating the documentation
  - Any omissions must be documented appropriately
  - Any additional information or patient assessment must be documented in the nursing notes
- Report
  - Any omissions
  - Patient response
  - Any interventions or further assessment and monitoring, outcomes and actions
  - Any potential or actual errors that may have occurred

Safe medicines management

Nurses are integral to safe medicine administration. This alone requires many stages of checking and understanding with regard to the patients, the prescription and the drug.

The NMC (2008) recommends that the checking alone should include the following:

- The patient's identity matches that on the prescription and that this is verified.
- The patient's knowledge is assessed with regard to their drug regimen, contra-indications, risks and benefits of the proposed medicine, and that these are explained to the patient in a way that they can understand and comprehend in order to agree to the treatment.
- The medicine has been clearly prescribed, including the dose and frequency.

- The medicine dispensed has been prepared and labelled accordingly, with an expiry date.

- The preparation of the medicine is clearly indicated and the information is from a reliable resource such as the British National Formulary (BNF); trust formulary/policy/guidelines; pharmacist or manufacturer recommendations.

- Any calculations in the dosage preparation, formulation and route are carried out by the nurse independently and checked with another health care professional and verified correct.

- Any equipment required to administer the medicine is clean, checked and in working order, and the nurse has had the required training to operate and use it safely.

- A non-touch technique is practised and infection risks are minimised at all times during medicine administration.

- Medicines are administered safely and appropriately at the patient's bedside without interruption, at the patient's pace and consumption/administration is verified.

- Documentation is completed accurately, timely and honestly to support actions taken or omitted.

- Monitoring and assessment of the patient and their response to the treatment is carried out during or after medicine administration and is documented and reported accordingly.

This is not an exhaustive list; however, it should complement your local policies and guidelines and NMC Standards for Medicine Management (NMC, 2008).

The approach to safe medicines management should reflect a systematic process, which will be further discussed in the next chapter. Additionally, nurses must have pharmacological knowledge and this will be addressed in Chapter 5.

The expanding role

Nurses today take on much greater responsibility than in the past. They have an active role in ordering diagnostic tests such as x-rays, performing diagnostic procedures such as endoscopies, actively managing patients from the perspective of making referrals, admission and discharge planning, managing patients' illnesses independently under agreed protocols, prescribing medications and treatments, consulting on pain management and other aspects of patient care pathways, leading nurse-led clinics, taking on key management positions, developing and implementing protocols and guidelines, triaging patients, performing advanced resuscitation skills and minor surgical procedures, leading outpatient departments and local health services, and leading nurses and the profession from political and senior leadership and management roles.

The advanced practitioner can be seen in a variety of specialist roles and is highly skilled, which can be seen as a strength but has also stretched the practitioner and their capabilities. In order to fulfil these specialist roles, critical decision-making skills, management skills, specialist knowledge and expertise are essential. The nurse's role has evolved and developed, as has technology and health care in the twenty-first century.

ACTIVITY 2.3

Consider the history of nursing and influential nurses of their time:

Florence Nightingale

Mary Seacole

Clara Barton

What were their contributions to nursing and how have these shaped where we are today?

....

....

....

....

....

....

Boundaries

In all areas of employment, nurses should be familiar with their job description and contract of employment, and have a sound awareness of their professional limitations and boundaries. This is essential to safe practice and reflective of one's accountability. Professional limitations are set out to protect both patients and practitioners.

Boundaries are important barriers, and a means of protection. It is vital that nurses and health care professionals reflect upon, consider and indeed discuss such boundaries. This gives rise to effective teamwork and a clear understanding of what one can and cannot do. It is important to realise, and to accept, that we cannot be everything to everyone, and that there are consequences for our actions.

ACTIVITY 2.4

Review your working contract and/or job description. What limitations are set for your practice?

....

....

....

....

Can you identify what your role and responsibilities entail?

....

....

....

....

Nurses undoubtedly can get caught up in multitasking and taking on 'too' much, but this lends itself to disaster, and would be largely unsupported by an employer if the boundaries and limitations are not respected and are overreached. In Chapter 1 your professional role was discussed, as were professional and legal implications and restrictions on your practice. Nurses need to be familiar with legislation that encompasses health and safety at work and protection for employees and employers.

ACTIVITY 2.5

Access the Office of Public Sector Information website at www.opsi.gov.uk. Locate legislation that addresses health and safety at work and identify your responsibilities as an employee and your employer's responsibilities.

....

....

....

....

....

....

In medicines management it is important that we follow guidelines for safe practice, that we understand our role and limitations, and that we share good practice and desist from practice that can lead to errors or patient harm. There is no shortcut to safe and effective care. It is important that everyone shares the responsibility and that this sharing is reflected in the teamwork and in our safe and effective delivery of care.

Chapter summary

All members of the inter-professional team are essential to and responsible for safe medicines management. Each has a unique role and together can incorporate effective teamwork through good communication and having a common goal – the patient's safety, management and care delivery.

All members of the inter-professional team have boundaries and are accountable for what they do and for what they do not do. It is important that we respect these boundaries and indeed our limitations. But, it is equally important that we work together as a team. Failure to do this will compromise the safety of the patient and could lead to an untoward event and indeed a preventable mistake – but this will be covered in the next chapter.

So what have you learned?

Let's do a quick check. Write down your answers to the following questions or simply tick whether the statement is true or false.

1. The inter-professional team is made up of many disciplines in health care. List all those that you recall from this chapter, or more that you have worked with.

   ....

   ....

   ....

   ....

2. Everyone that makes up the inter-professional team has the same goal.

   True ☐   False ☐

3. What are three characteristics of effective teamwork?

   ....

   ....

   ....

4. A job description can help to clarify our role and responsibilities and set boundaries for our practice.

   True ☐   False ☐

5. What is a limitation to your role as a nurse? Why is this important to understand?

....

....

....

....

....

....

References and key texts

Dimond, B. (ed.) (2008) *Legal Aspects of Nursing*, 5th edn. London: Pearson.

GMC (General Medical Council) (2010) *Members' Code of Conduct*. Available at http://www.gmc-uk.org

Health and Safety at Work Act (1974) London: HMSO.

NMC (Nursing and Midwifery Council) (2008) *Standards for Medicines Management*. London: NMC.

NMC (Nursing and Midwifery Council) (2010) *Nurse and Midwife Prescribing of Unlicensed Medicines*. Available at http://www.nmc-uk.org/Documents/Circulars/2010circulars/NMCcircular04_2010.pdf

RPSGB (Royal Pharmaceutical Society of Great Britain) (2007) *The Code of Ethics for Pharmacists and Pharmacy Technicians*. Available at http://www.rpsgb.org.uk

Additional reading

Audit Commission (2001) *A Spoonful of Sugar: Medicines Management in NHS Hospitals*. Wetherby: Audit Commission Publications.

Department of Health (2000) *The NHS Plan: A Plan for Investment, a Plan for Reform*. London: The Stationery Office.

Department of Health (2001) *The Expert Patient: A New Approach to Chronic Disease Management for the 21st Century*. London: The Stationery Office.

Department of Health (2002) *Developing Key Roles for Nurses and Midwives: A Guide for Managers*. London: The Stationery Office.

Department of Health (2002) *Liberating the Talents: Helping Primary Care Trusts and Nurses to Deliver the NHS Plan*. London: The Stationery Office.

Department of Health (2003) *Essence of Care: Patient-focused Benchmarks for Clinical Governance*. London: The Stationery Office.

Department of Health (2004) *Building a Safer NHS for Patients: Improving Medication Safety*. London: The Stationery Office.

Healthcare Commission (2007) *The Best Medicines: The Best Management of Medicines in Acute and Specialists Trusts*. London: Commission for Healthcare Audit and Inspection.

Hewitt-Taylor, J. (2002) 'Evidence-based practice'. *Nursing Standard* 17: 47–52.

Home Office (2007) *Independent Prescribing of Controlled Drugs by Nurse and Pharmacists Independent Prescribers*. Available at http://www.homeoffice.gov.uk

Hughes, S.L., Whittlesea, C. and Luscombe, D. (2002) 'Patients' knowledge and perceptions of the side-effects of OTC medication'. *Journal of Clinical Pharmacology and Therapeutics* 27: 243–8.

McKenna, H. (2005) 'Commentary: Dynamic effects on nursing roles with changing healthcare services'. *Journal of Research Nursing* 10: 99–106.

NMC (Nursing and Midwifery Council) (2006) *Standards of Proficiency for Nurse and Midwife Prescribers*. London: NMC.

NPSA (National Patient Safety Agency) (2007) *Safety in Doses: Improving the Use of Medicines in the NHS*. Available at http://npsa.uk/patientsafety/medication-zone/reviews-of-medication-incidents/.

Royal College of Nursing (2008) *Nursing Our Future: An RCN Study into the Challenges Facing Today's Nursing Students in the UK*. London: RCN.

Royal College of Nursing (2009) *Breaking Down the Barriers, Driving up the Standards: The Role of the Ward Sister and the Charge Nurse*. London: RCN.

Tschudin, V. (ed.) (2003) *Approaches to Ethics: Nursing Beyond Boundaries*. Edinburgh: Butterworth Heinemann.

Websites:

http://www.gmc-uk.org

http://www.homeoffice.gov.uk

http://www.nmc-uk.org

http://www.opsi.gov.uk

http://www.rpsgb.org.uk

Chapter 3

Safe systems

When you have completed this chapter you should:

- have an understanding of safe systems and the indications for this in medicines management
- understand the relevance and importance of organisations and government initiatives that aim to protect the public and how legislation supports safe systems
- be able to apply a safe approach to clinical practice of established routines and safety checks

Your starting point

Answer the following questions and begin reflecting on safe systems in medicines management.

1. Write down what you think it means to be 'safe'?

   ....

   ....

2. What key characteristics and skills must one have in order to 'be safe'?

   ....

   ....

3. Provide an example of a 'safe system' in your clinical practice.

   ....

   ....

4. Does this system reflect policy or guidelines or legislation?

   Yes ☐   No ☐   Unsure ☐

5. What is the first safety check that is fundamental in safe medicine administration?

   ....

   ....

6. Why are controlled drugs locked in a cupboard?

   ....

   ....

7. What legislation regulates medicines?

   ....

   ....

Introduction

This chapter looks at 'systems', which are an important element in medicines management. The systems approach is supported by research, as are the effective and safe systems of industry, health care organisations and clinical practice generally. A safe systems approach is central to medicines management and safe practice. Systematic approaches, or processes, encourage routine and safety checks – this way of working is not limited to health care but is seen in many industries and organisations. This chapter will focus on systems for safe practice in medicines management, building upon what you have learned in the previous chapter. Further, key government documents and organisations that play a vital role in developing safe systems of practice will be explored in this chapter as well as pertinent legislation.

Why do systems checks?

Let's first consider other professionals and how they work. Ask yourself what systems they adopt to ensure their actions are safe, and indeed systematic.

ACTIVITY 3.1

List the checks and responsibilities for

An airplane pilot and cabin crew before take-off: ....

....

....

A Formula One racing team: ....

....

....

Now compare this with the checks and responsibilities of a nurse in medicine administration. Do they differ? Are there similarities?

....

....

....

....

How we do things and the order in which we do them are important. Safe steps and checks should be imbedded into a routine. There is no place for shortcuts and each step is equally important.

> Consider what would happen if, for example, the pilot left out an important systems check before take-off? Or what if the racing team missed one tyre check? What if the name band wasn't checked before the patient was given a blood transfusion or if the bedside identification check was missed entirely?

System failures

In its 2003 annual report the Serious Hazards of Transfusion Steering Group (SHOT) identified that the most common error during blood transfusions was failure of the pre-transfusion bedside checking procedure, where, at the bedside check, nurses failed to detect an error earlier in the transfusion chain. Further analysis showed errors where expired units were infused, checking blood against documentation took place away from the bedside, identification wristbands were absent and in some cases complete omission of the bedside identification check occurred (SHOT, 2003).

Medication errors occur when human and system factors interact with the complex process of prescribing, dispensing and administering medicines. Many medication errors occur at 'handover points' within the health care system (Department of Health, 2004).

Strategies to improve systems include:

- Systems for reporting and learning from medication errors
- Recognising near misses as a failure in systems predisposing error

- Building error traps into the medication process
- Investigation and analysis of mistakes
- Education and training for safety
- Improved communications interface
- Formal structures for managing medication safety.

Key organisations and government bodies

Patient safety is dominated by government, research, legislation and guidance that aim to influence safe practice and encompass safe systems, particularly in medicines management. There are key organisations that have a direct impact on patient care and influence clinical practice, organisational policies and systems of safe practice.These are identified and explained below.

Department of Health

The Department of Health exists to improve the health and well-being of people in England. Its purpose is to provide health and social care policy, guidance and publications. It is responsible for health protection, health improvement and health inequality issues in England (Department of Health, 2010).

Medicines and Healthcare Products Regulatory Agency (MHRA)

The MHRA is the UK government agency responsible for ensuring that medicines and medical devices work and are acceptably safe. The agency was created in 2003 from the merger of the Medical Devices Agency and the Medicines Control Agency. It is responsible for the regulation of medicines and medical devices and equipment used in health care and the investigation of harmful incidents. It also looks after blood and blood products, working with UK blood services, health care providers, and other relevant organisations to improve blood quality and safety (MHRA, 2010).

National Institute for Health and Clinical Excellence (NICE)

NICE is an independent organisation responsible for providing national guidance on promoting good health and preventing and treating ill health (NICE, 2009). It produces guidance on a wide range of drugs and other technologies to support the cost-effective use of the NHS; it lists recommendations to improve the NHS and quality of care; and it holds various meetings that are open to the public and press in support of NICE's commitment to having processes in place that are rigorous, open and transparent. The guidance produced by NICE can improve care for patients and empower health professionals to deliver the most clinically effective and cost-effective care (NICE, 2009).

National Patient Safety Agency (NPSA)

The NPSA is part of the NHS with a mandate to identify patient safety issues and find appropriate solutions. It was established in 2003 and has led and contributed to improved, safe patient care by informing, supporting and influencing organisations and people working in the health sector. The three divisions, covering the UK health service, have key functions within the NHS: (1) National Reporting and Learning Service which aims to reduce risks to patients receiving NHS care and improve safety; (2) National Clinical Assessment Service which supports the resolution of concerns about the performance of individual clinical practitioners to help ensure their practice is safe and valued; (3) National Research Ethics Service which protects the rights, safety, dignity and well-being of research participants taking part in clinical trials and other research within the NHS.

Nursing and Midwifery Council (NMC)

The NMC is a UK organisation set up by Parliament to ensure that practitioners deliver a high standard of care. It exists to safeguard the health and well-being of the public. It sets standards for nurses and midwives to meet in their working lives; sets standards for education throughout nurses' and midwives' careers, after they initially qualify; and keeps a register of all nurses and midwives in the UK which is a legal requirement in order to work in the UK. It sets a code of conduct which all registrants are required to work within and adhere to. Nurses and midwives must provide proof that they fulfil the NMC requirements for keeping their skills and knowledge up to date.

Key documents on medicines management

The Department of Health report *Building a Safer NHS for Patients: Improving Medication Safety* (2004) highlights what is known with regard to the frequency, nature and causes of medication errors. It recommends models of good practice, and provides solutions and interventions through national and local strategies.

ACTIVITY 3.2

Access the Department of Health website at www.doh.gov.uk and locate this report. Identify three key recommendations for safer practice in medicines management.

There are numerous reports that have collectively set the agenda for redesigning pharmaceutical services for patients, to improve safety and quality of care.

ACTIVITY 3.3

Using the web links below, access the following documents and identify how these support 'safe systems'. Jot down some notes below.

(a) www.npsa.nhs.uk *Safety in Doses: Improving the Use of Medicines in the NHS* (NPSA, 2009)

(b) www.dh.gov.uk *Building a Safer NHS for Patients: Improving Medication Safety* (Department of Health, 2004)

(c) www.mhra.gov.uk *Medicines and Medical Devices Regulation: What You Need to Know* (MHRA, 2008)

(d) www.nmc-uk.org *Standards for Medicines Management* (NMC, 2008)

....

....

....

....

....

....

A systems approach to safe medication

The Department of Health identifies that a systems approach accepts that humans are fallible and that mistakes can happen. They can be expected to occur – and may occur regardless of the competence of individuals working within the system. A systems approach therefore focuses on the conditions under which individuals work rather than the individual, and on understanding how these conditions can predispose to errors.

For nurses, systems are a key asset in error prevention, as their checks may be the 'final' check in an inter-professional chain of prescribing, dispensing, administering.

A commonsense approach requires three checks in three steps:

1. *Bedside check* – This check must come first! At this check, if the patient does not have an identity wristband this has to be rectified immediately. If the prescription is not checked against the patient details first, then potentially it may be the wrong prescription for that patient.

2. *Prescription check* – This includes the Five Rights (see Chapter 4) and reading the prescription in its entirety before medicines are prepared, mixed and given.

3. *Documentation check* – Documenting once the patient has taken the medicine is the final step. This should occur once the nurse has verified that the patient has taken the medicine. A common

error in practice, as a result of a 'hurry-up' attitude, is to leave medicines at the patient's bedside, not witness the patient consume the medicine and to document that it has occurred before it has happened. This is unsafe!

What do you think are the possible dangers of this?

ACTIVITY 3.4

Go to the NMC website at www.nmc-uk.org and access the guidance on records and record keeping. You may wish to jot down some notes below.

....

....

....

....

....

....

The Department of Health (2004) identifies 'person and systems' approaches to medication error (Figure 3.1).

This approach looks at both individuals and systems and it is important to recognise the causes of error and our reaction. It is helpful to have systems in place such as adapting the Five Rights or recognising that we all have a responsibility to check, and effectively minimise error. Reason (1997) identifies a 'Swiss cheese' model of error prevention where each layer is defence against medication error. This includes checking by the pharmacist; the prescriber; at the time of administration; effective communication between health care professionals and the patient at each stage. However, he also identifies that there are holes in the system (hence the cheese), but increasing the layers can reduce the chance of error (Reason, 1997).

Thus we can see how teamwork, effective communication and a systematic approach can help to reduce error, minimise risk and ensure safe practice in medicines management. Practice that demonstrates a well-designed system with built-in safeguards is safer – and this includes *meaningful* checks.

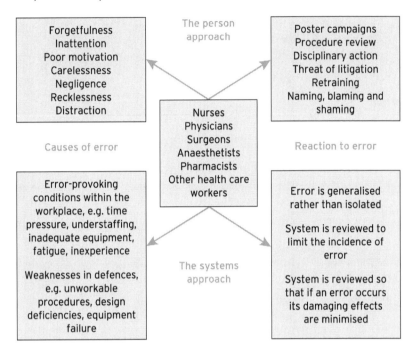

Figure 3.1 **The person and systems approaches to medication error**
Source: Department of Health, 2004, figure 2.4, p. 31

Within any system it is imperative that we learn from our mistakes in order to prevent their recurrence. This requires vigilance, reporting near-misses and potential errors, sharing and modelling good practice and adopting those systems and recommendations that we know to be effective in minimising harm and risk to patients.

Key legislation on medicines and drugs

For nurses in clinical practice, the process of administering medicines is a result of legal and professional developments and legislative powers. Parliament is the highest law maker in the English legal system and gives rise to much of the legislation that governs society. Health care is equally influenced by legislation and therefore it is important to understand those statutory instruments that have an influence on how we act, how we are governed and indeed how we are protected at work. Chapter 1 provided an overview of the English legal system and relevant law, which will not be repeated in this chapter; rather, key legislation will be examined in the context of nursing.

Licensing is necessary for all medicines before their use by the public, as a means of ensuring safe standards. Pharmaceutical companies must adhere to regulations in their development, testing and clinical trials, research and marketing of all drugs to be used by the consumer. Regulatory agencies therefore play a role in granting licences and the law is needed as a compulsory measure to ensure all medicines are indeed licensed before their use.

It is not only use but also the manufacture, distribution, storage and supply of medicines that are governed by statutory instruments. These have an impact on assessment, indication and use and control of medicines used in health care.

Key legislation that pertains to medicines include:

- Medicines Act 1968
- Misuse of Drugs Act 1971
- Health Act 2006
- The Medicines (Pharmacies) (Responsible Pharmacist) Regulations 2008
- Medicinal Products: Prescription by Nurses Act 1992
- Consumer Protection Act 1987
- Sales of Goods Act 1979

ACTIVITY 3.5

Of the listed legislation governing medicines, select one and access this via the web link www.opsi.gov. Jot down some notes below.

What you have probably noticed is the complexity and length of such statutory instruments. Thus an understanding of how these come into force and are applied to everyday practice is important.

Let's look first at regulations and laws relating to drug use in practice. There are three key pieces of legislation that address issues such as drug packaging, labelling and storage; production, use and supply; possession; scheduling and classification of controlled substances (see Table 3.1).

Table 3.1 **Key legislation**

Legislation	Remit
Medicines Act 1968	Licensing system for medicines manufacture, distribution, prescription, supply, packaging and labelling
Misuse of Drugs Act 1971	Regulations governing production, supply and possession of controlled drugs (CDs) to prevent their use and controls to forfeit, search and arrest
Misuse of Drugs Regulations (MDR 2001)	Schedules drugs according to the different level of control required (CDs are subject to the highest level)

The *Medicines Act* was originally passed by Parliament in 1968 and has since had amended directions. It is largely responsible for a classification system for public use of medicines but also covers many different aspects of their use. The three classifications are P, GSL and POM.

- *Pharmacy-only* (P) are those medicines that can be sold to the consumer under the supervision and direction of a pharmacist in registered premises such as a pharmacy, whether this be independent or in a grocery supermarket. Such medicines do not require a prescription and are often referred to as 'over the counter' from a pharmacist. They would not be those medicines found on the shelves stocked in your local shop or supermarket. Controls are based upon packaging and content, quantity/dosage and formulation.

- *General sales list* (GSL) are those medicines the consumer can purchase in a local shop or supermarket without supervision but have controls based upon packaging and content, quantity/dosage and formulation.

● *Prescription-only medicines* (POMs) are those medicines that can only be obtained with a prescription from an authorised prescriber or GP. They could not be obtained otherwise.

These controls for the consumer are for good reason and act as a means of protection and control.

The *Misuse of Drugs Act 1971* schedules those drugs that we associate with misuse and addiction, such as cocaine, diamorphine (heroin), methadone and morphine. These fall under strict rules of compliance, use and control and are kept under lock and key. Legislation is necessary to prevent their misuse. The law enforcement powers associated with controlled drugs (CDs) include search, forfeiture and arrest. It is essential therefore that when we consider the policy and guidelines associated with controlled drugs and their use in practice, we as nurses adhere to these policies and strict controls. Health care professionals are not above the law!

ACTIVITY 3.6

Review your local policy on controlled drugs and list those steps that you must follow when preparing, mixing and administering a controlled drug such as Oramorph 10 mg.

....

....

....

....

....

....

Are there any limitations as to who has responsibility for the keys to the CD cupboard?

....

....

Along with the NMC standards of care (NMC, 2008) and your professional duty of care, which were discussed in more detail in Chapter 1, there are further key statutory instruments that aim to protect the public, the consumer and indeed you, the employee.

Nurses have to be aware of the law with respect to consumers and the public where medicines management, equipment and fitness for purpose are concerned. It is essential that we as professionals are able to work in an environment that is safe, and that processes are in place to ensure our safety, not only from a physical perspective but also in terms of risk assessment, policy and procedures that guide safe practice. Table 3.2 identifies legislation that aims to protect the public and the consumer, and to educate patients in medicines management.

Table 3.2 Consumer legislation on the provision and use of medicines

Legislation	Remit
EU Directive 92/27/EEC 1999	Drug information to be provided to patients
Health Act 2009	Contains provisions on a range of policies regarding quality and delivery of NHS services
Consumer Protection Act 1987	Covers product liability, consumer safety and pricing issues and extends its powers to imported medicines
Sale of Goods Act 1979	Covers goods for sale, their use and fitness for purpose

In addition, nurses need to consider their health and safety at work and legislation that helps to protect them while at work.

Chapter summary

A key component of the nurse's role requires an understanding of 'safe systems' management, elements of medicine administration and the effectiveness in care delivery. For nurses, this is fundamental to their role, where relevant knowledge, skill and expertise are necessary. It is the very essence of what nurses do and who they are, in defining safe and effective patient care and standards of care.

The process of medicines management revolves around outcomes and indicators of patient care, evidence-based research and systems development for patient safety and medication use and administration.

Collectively it requires knowledge and appreciation of pharmacological principles and associated complexities of the biological sciences. It requires understanding of the processes of medication, their storage and use, therapeutic indications and contra-indications, administration, monitoring and documentation and overall effective and competent management. It requires nurses to reflect on practice and continue to develop new skills and enhance their practice in order to meet the challenges of safe delivery of patient care and effective medicines management.

Health care organisations are increasingly becoming aware of the importance of safe medication practice and issues in relation to medicines management. As a result, recommendations for reducing the risks of medication incidents have led to the implementation and use of dedicated procedures of an organisation-wide management system to address medication safety. This involves procedures that include regular review of incident reports, actions by multidisciplinary groups and publication of summary reports of progress in reducing these risks.

It is clear that in order for this management system to be effective, reporting of errors has to occur so that we can learn from mistakes and put systems into place to reduce further incidence. But what if mistakes and incidents go unreported or undetected? Not all medication errors result in death. And not all practitioners or patients may be aware that an error or mistake has occurred. This will be explored in greater detail in the next chapter.

So what have you learned?

Let's do a quick check. Write down your answers to the following questions or simply tick whether the statement is true or false.

1. The Department of Health provides health and social care policy, guidance and publications.

   True ☐   False ☐

2. List two essential checks in a safe systems approach to minimising error and ensuring safe practice.

....

....

3. Drug information must be provided to patients as a result of what legislative instrument? (Choose A, B or C)

A. Health Act 2006 ☐
B. EU Directive 92/27/EEC 1999 ☐
C. Medicines Act 1968 ☐

4. What is the difference between pharmacy-only and prescription-only medicines?

....

....

5. Which agency is responsible for ensuring that medicines and medical devices work and are acceptably safe?

....

References and key texts

Department of Health (2004) *Building a Safer NHS for Patients: Improving Medication Safety*. London: The Stationery Office.

Department of Health (2010) *How to Use Essence of Care: Best Practice Guidelines*. Available at http://www.dh.gov.uk/en/Publicationsandstatistics/Publications/PublicationsPolicyAndGuidance/DH_119969.

MHRA (Medicines and Healthcare Products Regulatory Agency) (2008) *Medicines and Medical Devices Regulation: What You Need to Know*. Available at http://www.mhra.gov.uk/NewsCentre/CON203173.

MHRA (Medicines and Healthcare Products Regulatory Agency) (2010) *Medical Device Alert: Medical Devices in General and Non-Medical Products*. Available at http://www.mhra.gov.uk/Publications/Safetywarnings/MedicalDeviceAlerts/CON065771.

NICE (National Institute for Health and Clinical Excellence) (2009) *Medicines Adherence Guidelines*. Available at http://www.nice.org.uk/nicemedia/live/11766/43042/43042.pdf

NMC (Nursing and Midwifery Council) (2008) *Standards for Medicines Management*. London: NMC.

NPSA (National Patient Safety Agency) (2003) *Annual Report*. Available at http://www.npsa.nhs.uk/170_annual_report_2002_2003.pdf.inc.

NPSA (National Patient Safety Agency) (2004) *Seven Steps to Patient Safety: An Overview Guide for NHS Staff*. Available at http://www.npsa.co.uk/patientsafety/improving patient safety/7 steps/.

NPSA (National Patient Safety Agency) (2007) *Safety in Doses: Improving the Use of Medicines in the NHS*. Available at http://npsa.uk/patientsafety/medication-zone/reviews-of-medication-incidents/.

NPSA (National Patient Safety Agency) (2009) *Safety in Doses: Improving the Use of Medicines in the NHS*. Available at http://www.nrls.npsa.nhs.uk/resources/patient-safety-topics/medication-safety/.

Reason, J. (1997) *Managing the Risks of Organisational Accidents*. Aldershot: Ashgate.

SHOT (Serious Hazards of Transfusion Steering Group) (2003) *SHOT Report*. Available at http://www.shotuk.org/shot-reports/reports-and-summaries-2003/.

Additional reading

Audit Commission (2001) *A Spoonful of Sugar: Medicines Management in NHS Hospitals*. Wetherby: Audit Commission Publications.

Department of Health (2002) *Advisory Council on the Misuse of Drugs Report: The Classification of Cannabis under the Misuse of Drugs Act 1971*. London: The Stationery Office.

Department of Health (2007) *Safer Management of Controlled Drugs: Early Action*. London: The Stationery Office.

Dougherty, L. and Lister, S. (2008) *Royal Marsden Hospital Manual of Clinical Nursing Procedures*. Oxford: Wiley Blackwell.

Healthcare Commission (2007) *The Best Medicines: The Management of Medicines in Acute and Specialist Trusts*. London: Commission for Healthcare Audit and Inspection.

Hughes, S.L., Whittlesea, C. and Luscombe, D. (2002) 'Patient's knowledge and perceptions of the side-effects of OTC medication'. *Journal of Clinical Pharmacology and Therapeutics* 27: 243–8.

Jordan, S., Tunnicliffe, C. and Sykes, A. (2002) 'Minimising side effects: the clinical impact of nurse administration "side effects" check list'. *Journal of Advanced Nursing* 37: 155–65.

Wilson, D. and DeVito, T.P. (2004) 'The sixth right of medication administration'. *Nurse Educator* 29: 131–2.

Websites

http://audit-commission.gov.uk

http://www.dh.gov.uk

http://www.mhra.gov.uk

http://www.nice.org.uk

http://www.nmc-uk.org

http://www.npsa.nhs.uk

http://www.opsi.gov.uk

Chapter 4

Errors in medicines management and their prevention

When you have completed this chapter you should:

- understand what constitutes an 'error'
- have an awareness of poor practice or unsafe practice that can lead to a mistake
- be able to review types of errors and their causes in medicines management
- understand how to report and prevent error and improve patient safety in medicines management

Your starting point

Answer the following questions and begin reflecting on instances in practice where a mistake may have occurred or an error resulted.

1. Write the definition of

   Error: ....

   ....

   Mistake: ....

   ....

2. Are there any similarities in the two definitions you have given in question 1?

   ....

3. List three types of error that can occur in practice in medicines management.

   ....

   ....

   ....

4. Choose one of your answers in question 3. Write down how you think this can be prevented from occurring.

   ....

   ....

   ....

   ....

   ....

Introduction

Mistakes or errors can be the result of one or more contributing factors, but more often than not they happen as a result of poor or unsafe practice, or as a result of system failure. In Chapter 1 we discussed negligence and acts that were described as 'careless' which could result in patient harm. That is the danger of a mistake. There should be no doubt in your mind that a strong link exists between patient harm and mistakes. It is important to understand that by increasing awareness this can help to decrease error incidence. Often it is only when something goes wrong, that we realise a mistake occurred (Dimond, 2008), and consequences of this are unfortunate. The outcome of our mistake as a result of poor judgement, lack of knowledge or unsafe practice leads to patient harm. This is unacceptable. A better awareness and learning from mistakes can prevent them from recurring.

Mistakes – what are they and why do they happen?

'I think I may have given Mr Kemp's medicine to Mr Kean by mistake'

'I thought I set the infusion pump at 50 ml/hr – I cannot understand how the infusion has finished already!'

'8 tablets seems a lot to give at once, doesn't it?'

'I am sure you give an intramuscular injection about . . . around . . . er . . . here'

It might be easier to explain how to prevent mistakes from occurring than to explain why they happen in the first instance. But first, we need to understand what they are and why they occur.

There are several words used to describe essentially the same thing – a mistake, an error, wrongdoing, a clinical incident. The word 'error' comes from the Latin word *errare*, meaning 'to stray, to err'. By definition an *error is a mistake*. It is defined as 'the state or condition

63

of being wrong in conduct or in judgement'. A mistake can take many forms but for the purpose of this book and its intention, the focus will be in medicines management. Therefore a definition for medication error will be necessary.

The above quotes from nurses may have helped you to determine what constitutes a mistake. In medicines management, mistakes are a grave concern; every day about 2.5 million medicines are prescribed across the UK, and although most medicines are used safely, sometimes errors occur which can lead to harm.

A working definition

The National Patient Safety Agency defines a medication error as

> 'an incident in which there has been an error in the process of pre-scribing, dispensing, preparing, administering, monitoring, or providing medicine advice, regardless of whether any harm occurred.'
>
> (NPSA, 2007)

The cost of errors to the NHS is great and the effect on patients can be devastating. Medication errors can cause unnecessary pain and harm to patients and can lead to death – they account for a substantial strain on NHS resources at an estimated cost of £400 million a year (NHSLA, 2008).

The majority of medication incidents reported have been related to the administration of medicines, followed by incidents related to the preparation, dispensing and prescribing of medicines. The most common types of medication incidents reported and the most frequently occurring type of medication error include the wrong dose, the wrong strength or frequency, omission and the wrong medicine. Together these account for over half of all medication incidents reported (NPSA, 2007).

So why do errors occur?

Both the administration of medicines and the expanding role of the nurse introduce complexity and uncertainty in our practice to such a degree that there is an inherent risk to patients. Often it is only after an error has happened that we are even aware of it, if at all. The burden of an error is great and the emotion unimaginable. The error is often the result of carelessness, lack of regard or the result of a mistake that did not have to happen. Most errors and mistakes are highly preventable. Every day, approximately 2.5 million medicines are prescribed to patients in hospitals and the community (NPSA, 2007), and although most medicines are used safely and effectively, sometimes errors happen that can lead to harm to patients.

ACTIVITY 4.1

Below are two columns. On the left is a common type of error, on the right is a space for you to write a definition or provide an example of what this error is.

Error	Definition or example
Wrong patient	
Omission	
Monitoring	
Wrong medicine	
Incorrect time	
Wrong route	
Wrong preparation	
Wrong formulation	

Types of error

Omission errors

Although omitting a medicine is a commonly reported error, it is not always considered a serious error. However, where the medicine is considered vital for the patient, such as medicines used to treat epilepsy or to prevent strokes, omission can lead to permanent harm or death.

Patient identification errors

At any stage in the medication process, medicines intended for one patient can be given to another patient in error, and often this is due to incorrect patient identification. Almost 5 per cent of reported medication incidents relate to mismatching between patients and medicines (NPSA, 2007). In some instances the administration of a drug incompatible with a patient's diagnosis may be given. Matching of patients with their care is central to improving patient safety; however, three main types of error that typically involve the patient being wrongly identified are:

1. A patient is given the wrong treatment as a result of a failure to match them correctly with samples, specimens or x-rays.

2. A patient is given the wrong treatment as a result of a failure in communication between staff or because 'checking procedures' were not performed correctly.

3. A patient is given treatment intended for another patient as a result of a failure to identify him or her correctly.

Examples of such errors include:

- Mrs Johns' blood, tissue sample or specimen is confused with Mrs Jones', leading to one or, possibly, both receiving the wrong diagnosis and/or wrong treatment.

- A patient is incorrectly operated on – for example the wrong limb is amputated or the wrong kidney removed – because of a failure in communication between staff and checking procedures.

- Mr U. Patel is given the medicines intended for Mr V. Patel.

ACTIVITY 4.2

How could you have prevented the three errors listed above?

In addition, for some groups of patients (such as children) and in some settings (such as general practice), medication error was the most commonly reported type of incident. Vulnerable patients include children up to the age of 4, who have been identified as having the second-highest percentage of medication incidents of all age groups, after patients in the over-75 age group (NPSA, 2007).

Prescribing errors

A prescribing error can occur from a prescribing decision or from the prescription-writing process and results in an unintentional but significant reduction in the probability of treatment being timely and effective. It may also result in increased risk of harm compared with generally accepted practice.

Examples of this type of error include:

1. Prescribing without taking into account the patient's clinical status
2. Failure to communicate essential information for the prescription
3. Transcription errors.

ACTIVITY 4.3

Can you provide an example of a prescribing error?

....

....

Dispensing errors

Although dispensing errors have a lower error rate, they do occur. The incidence is lower simply because this is where the majority of errors are in fact identified and this takes place *before* the medicine leaves the pharmacy. However, in the community, the most common dispensing errors include:

1. Incorrect strength of the medicine
2. Incorrect medicine.

ACTIVITY 4.4

Can you provide an example of a dispensing error?

....

....

Dispensing errors in hospitals account for a relatively small amount of events that result in harm – only one in five in relation to commonly dispensed medications, which include: prednisolone, morphine sulphate, isosorbide monitrate, warfarin, aspirin, lisinopril, carbamazepine, diclofenac, co-codamol, flucloxacillin. Only one-third of these erroneous medicines resulted in severe harm. The most common error was the wrong strength being dispensed.

ACTIVITY 4.5

Of the list of medicines provided above, choose three that you are unfamiliar with and complete the table below. You will need to access a resource such as the British National Formulary, http://bnf.org.uk.

Classification	Indication	Normal dosage	Route(s)	Side effects	Contra-indication(s)

This information will be revisited in further detail in Chapter 5.

Administration errors

Typically, nurses administer medicines within the inpatient setting where the rate of error can range anywhere from 3.5 to 50 per cent. This reflects a wide range of medication errors, typically 'wrong-time errors' where the medicine is administered correctly but not within the time period prescribed. Also, higher rates of error are associated with intravenous medicines as compared with oral medicines. This will be looked at in more detail:

- *Wrong medicine* - Often this type of error is associated with medicines whose names look alike or sound alike, where there may be confusion of medicines with similar names or mis-selection. In addition, errors can arise from medicines having similar names and similar packaging.
- *Incorrect dosage* - This type of error may be due to a mislabelled package or to a dose calculation error which results in the patient receiving perhaps ten times too much drug.
- *Wrong formulation* - These errors can occur when medicines are prepared in the wrong form. Of the medication incidents analysed by the NPSA (2007), 2.4 per cent involved the right medicine being given in the wrong form.
- *Wrong route* - The incidents reported involved, for example, medicines intended to be given orally, mistakenly being given by injection. Wrong-route incidents with particular potential for severe harm involved the prescription or administration of a medicine by a different route from its licensed use.

Example 4.1 Giving a drug incorrectly can lead to patient harm

A patient was prescribed omeprazole N/G (via a nasogastric tube). The dose was prepared in a syringe. The drug was administered via a vascular access device rather than the nasogastric tube.

The patient became bradycardic and hypotensive but was resuscitated and recovered without immediate ill effect.

Monitoring errors

Monitoring errors are increasingly important because of the rising numbers of patients with chronic and multiple conditions which require careful management, specifically those patients that may have repeat prescriptions or where blood test monitoring and laboratory investigations may be needed in order to assess the dose required.

> Example 4.2
>
> An example of how this can lead to an error would be the failure to monitor a patient's blood pressure, heart rate and electrolytes which could lead to severe harm in patients with hypertension and heart failure and who are prescribed diuretics.

Let's take a moment to consider some of these conditions, so you can understand the importance of monitoring.

Blood pressure monitoring

This is indicated when giving anti-hypertensives or other cardiac medications that can have a direct effect on how the heart pumps, conduction, pressure and output. It is important to monitor the patient's normal blood pressure and watch for any signs of hypertension or hypotension.

Heart rate monitoring

This is indicated when giving medications that may cause bradycardia or tachycardia or cause cardiac arrhythmias. There are some drugs that can decrease the heart rate – digoxin, atropine – and others that can excite the cardiac muscle and increase the heart rate – adrenaline.

Electrolyte monitoring

Electrolytes are naturally occurring elements within the body which can alter when the normal homeostasis and hydration of the body become out of sync, perhaps through dehydration or hypervolemia. The administration of intravenous fluids, such as 0.09 per cent sodium chloride, can cause a shift within intracellular and extracellular spaces and affect electrolyte levels. Sometimes patients are prescribed potassium or calcium supplements which may also have an effect on the natural serum levels of potassium and calcium in the body. Diuretic therapy has a direct effect on the kidneys and may increase urine output, which may also have an adverse effect on electrolyte balance.

ACTIVITY 4.6

If a patient has an allergy to penicillin, which drug would you give? Tick as many or as few as you wish.

Augmentin ☐

Gentamicin ☐

Ampicillin ☐

Flucloxacillin ☐

Clarithromycin ☐

Clindamycin ☐

Erythromycin ☐

Cefuroxime ☐

Ceftriaxone ☐

Vancomycin ☐

Amoxicillin ☐

Incidents of patients being prescribed, dispensed or administered a medicine to which they are known to be allergic can account for about 3 per cent of all reported medication incidents in hospitals (NPSA, 2007).

Children are potentially more vulnerable

Recurring themes in medication incidents involving children include calculation errors; tenfold dose errors; problems with injectable medicines and the use of specific medicines such as gentamicin; and children being treated in non-paediatric areas.

Emphasis on reducing risks to children include using dedicated medicines on paediatric wards for children and using software to help calculate dosages for children based on body weight.

Example 4.3

A baby weighing 1600 g was prescribed a daily dose of 16.4 mg of an antibiotic. The dose should have been 8 mg per kg, equivalent to 12.8 mg for this baby. The error was discovered and rectified by the pharmacist before any doses were given.

ACTIVITY 4.7

Consider for a moment what it would feel like if you were a patient and you were given too much of a medication or given the wrong medication altogether. How would you feel?

....

....

....

....

....

....

Error prevention

If we can look at the mistakes made, often we identify what went wrong or how a weakness in the process led to the error. Targeting this is the first step towards error prevention. The topic of 'safe systems' has been addressed in the previous chapter, so this discussion will focus on safety, which includes reviewing the *process* of safe medicines management and tips for safe practice.

If we think back to the responsibilities of everyone involved in medicines management, we can see how the medication process comprises many steps and a series of stages that targets the inter-professional team:

1. *Prescribing* - involves the prescribing of a given medicine and dose.

2. *Dispensing* – involves supplying medicines to individuals or to hospital wards.

3. *Preparation* – involves preparing a dose of medicine for administration.

4. *Administration* – involves administering the dose by the appropriate route and method to the patient.

5. *Ingestion* – this is the patient taking the medication.

6. *Recording* – requires documentation that the medicine has been given.

7. *Monitoring* – involves checking the administration and effect of a medicine.

8. *Reporting* – requires communication to members of the health care team about the effectiveness of the medicine in relation to the patient's treatment and care.

9. *Reviewing* – involves regular review of the medication regimen so that medicines are adjusted, reordered or discontinued.

Errors can occur at *any* stage of the medication process and research has shown that the types and rate of errors vary at different stages. For example, in the first stage, errors can occur in the prescription and this can lead to further problems and increase the incidence of error.

Nurses, however, have a fundamental role in the third, and what could be the final, stage before the patient takes the medicine – because they are the third and final check. This has been shown to be an essential checkpoint and can minimise the chance of error.

Medication administration is an important and fundamental aspect of health care and a key nursing function that requires skilful, knowledgeable and competent performance *each and every time*. It is a skill that is performed by nearly *all* practising nurses and has a major influence on patient well-being. Therefore any deficiency in these expert and distinct skills can result in inaccurate medication administration and errors.

Let's review the process of administering medications, from the viewpoint of the nurse.

ACTIVITY 4.8

This is your prescription. Write down at least six steps, in chronological order, that you would take in administering this to your patient.

Drug: Paracetamol
Dose: 1 gram
Route: orally
Frequency: every 4–6 hours   due at 0800, 1200, 1800, 2200
Signed: Dr J. Dandy   Date: 10-10-10   Pharmacist initials: DT
Comments: Not to exceed 4 grams in a 24 hour period

....

....

....

....

....

....

....

....

....

....

....

....

Now, let's compare this to the list of steps below. How many from your list are the same as in the list below *and* in the same order?

Remember, each step requires knowledge, detailed procedures and skill.

1. The nurse checks the patient's identity to ensure the prescription card matches the patient's name, date of birth, hospital number.

2. The nurse ensures that the medications prescribed are for this patient and the prescription reflects the needs of the patient based upon their condition and diagnosis, medical history, age, weight and care plan.

3. The nurse checks whether the patient has taken this medication before and if he is familiar with the drug.

4. The nurse verifies whether the patient has any allergies, if this has been documented on the prescription chart.

5. The nurse verifies with the patient whether he understands why the drug is prescribed, what it is for and explains any side effects it may cause, in order for the patient to provide consent.

6. The nurse checks the prescription to ensure it is the correct drug prescribed for the correct time, dose and route.

7. The nurse obtains the medicine and checks the name and expiry date against the prescription chart.

8. The nurse checks the correct dosage and calculates the correct dose to administer; the stock dose is 500 mg therefore 2 tablets are required for a prescribed dose of 1 gram.

9. The tablets are dispensed into a clean medication cup using a non-touch sterile technique.

10. The nurse checks the dose, number of tablets, name of drug, expiry date, before replacing the medicine stock in either the patient's locker or drug trolley.

11. The nurse returns to the patient's bedside with the medication and informs the patient that she is offering a glass of water to take the paracetamol tablets, and observes the patient swallowing the tablets.

12. The nurse washes her hands.

13. The nurse documents the date, time, and dosage taken, and signs this on the prescription card.

14. The nurse returns to the patient within the hour to assess the patient (take his temperature or assess his pain, confirms the patient has not developed a rash).

ACTIVITY 4.9

Let's review what we should know about paracetamol. Complete the following chart. (You may need to access the BNF or other resource for the information.)

Classification: ....

....

Indication: ....

....

Dosage(s) and route(s):

....

....

....

....

....

Maximum dosage in 24 hours: ....

Calculation for the prescribed dose of 1 gram where the stock dose is 500 mg tablets

1 gram = 1000 mg

.... Each tablet is 500 mg therefore $500 \times 2 = 1000$

(Your answer should be: 2 tablets)

Side effects: ....

....

....

....

Cautions/contra-indications:

....

....

....

Nurses have a professional obligation to administer medications safely to patients. This is reflected in the NMC standards, which state that

> 'the administration of medicines is an important aspect of the professional practice of persons whose names are on the Council's register. It is not solely a mechanistic task to be performed in strict compliance with the written prescription of a medical practitioner. It requires thought and the exercise of professional judgement.'   (NMC, 2008b)

It is essential that practitioners who are responsible for the management and delivery of care to patients, particularly in medication management and administration, are aware of safe standards of practice and provisions and guidance set by the NMC with regard to medicines management. It is equally important to be aware of any local policies or guidelines for your practice in medicine administration pertinent to your role.

ACTIVITY 4.10

Access the NMC website at www.nmc-uk.org and locate the NMC *Standards for Medicines Management* (2008b). List those sections that are you consider essential to the safe administration of medicines.

Of the 10 sections there are 26 standards identified, *all* of which nurses and midwives have a responsibility to follow.

Section 1: Methods of supplying and/or administration of medicines

Section 2: Dispensing

Section 3: Storage and transportation

Section 4: Standards for practice of administration of medicines

ACTIVITY 4.11

Reflect on your answer to Activity 4.10 and the contents list above. How often do you incorporate these standards into your own clinical practice?

....

....

In administering any medication, assisting or overseeing any self-administration, nurses are required to exercise professional judgement, competence and expertise.

ACTIVITY 4.12

What do you think is meant by 'professional judgement'?

....

....

....

....

For example, in the scenario in Activity 4.8 where paracetamol is prescribed, would you give this drug if the patient: (tick all that would apply)

A. had renal failure ☐

B. had a fever ☐

C. had developed a slight rash the last time he took the drug ☐

D. could not swallow ☐

E. told you he was not in pain ☐

F. refused ☐

The above Activity is an example of demonstrating professional judge-ment based on what you know about this drug, about your patient, and your knowledge, skill and expertise. Remember, the patient trusts you with their health and well-being.

Knowledge in medication management and administration requires you to *understand* key principles in relation to the prescription, the patient and the drug. It is also essential that nurses have a general knowledge of pharmacological principles, which will be reviewed in the next chapter.

Some additional points

Self-administration and administration by carers
This is supported by the NMC; however, principles of safety, storage and security must be adhered to and local policies and procedures should be in place to support this. This includes precautions such as temperature control, exposure to light, locked storage and access.

Complementary and alternative therapies
These are becoming increasingly used in the treatment of patients and clients (NMC, 2004; Kelly et al., 2005). The appropriateness of the therapy to the condition of the patient or client and any coexisting treatments must be considered. Administration of these treatments must be carried out by specifically trained practitioners, with the patient's/client's consent, and practitioners should adhere to local policies and procedures in place to support and guide this treatment.

Tips for safe practice

The Five Rights

For many of us, safe practice is the process and application of what is often referred to as the 'Five Rights'. However, there could indeed be more, and it has been suggested that there are eight, nine, even twelve rights or steps that should be applied, in order to administer medicines safely. Whatever the number of steps, there must be consistency in applying a systematic approach which guides us in our practice and allows us to mentally, physically and indeed verbally go through a checking system in the safe administration of medicines to patients.

> **THE FIVE RIGHTS**
>
> The right patient
>
> The right drug
>
> The right dose
>
> The right route
>
> The right time

Following this alone is not without risk to the patient. In addition, there are external events that have a direct effect on the act of administering medicines and the outcome of safety. Time constraints, staff shortages, interruption, complex medicines and complex prescriptions, patient questioning, education and consent, and the time required to do this efficiently and safely are against us. In most instances it is the lack of time, that leaves nurses feeling rushed, taking short cuts and perhaps not being as thorough as we should. All of these reasons are a result of the system failing.

Calculation tips

Your experience of maths is personal and you have probably learned in a unique and different way from another person, perhaps the nurse you are working with now.

It is important that you understand the prescription and the calculation involved and *how* to get the correct answer - and that you *both* get the same answer.

Working out the correct dose is often about problem solving and taking 'steps' to solve some intermediate calculations:

- Look at the prescription and ask yourself what is required - what do you need to calculate?

- Break this down into smaller steps. For example, a metric conversion might be step one, as in the paracetamol example above. Step two may require multiplying or dividing.

- You may find a helpful formula to calculate the dosage, i.e.

  what you want (prescribed dose) ÷ what you have (stock dose)

- Finally, check that your answer makes sense . . . Would you realistically give 5 tablets or more at any one time?

- If you are going to use a calculator, first try to work out the answer in your head, then use the calculator to double check your answer. A false sense of reliance on any equipment is dangerous – know how to use the calculator first!

The Department of Health (2004) recommends that particular attention should be paid to checking the accuracy of complex dosage calculations. The NMC (2008b) recommends that calculations are performed independently then checked by two health care professionals.

Other measures for error prevention

Not all errors are a result of negligent practice; a variety of circumstances can lead to a professional making an error. These include inadequate training, lack of supervision, lack of support, staff shortages, unsatisfactory work conditions, limited resources and low morale (Department of Health, 2004). It is not just the individual that is culpable, but the system too may be to blame. It is true that every human can make mistakes and that we are not infallible. However, the problem that doctors and nurses face is that any error of judgement on their part, however inadvertent, can have fatal consequences or lead to suffering.

The consequence of such errors may result in little or no harm, but can nevertheless be distressing for patients and adversely affect the confidence of patients and staff. It has been identified that just under 10 per cent of hospital admissions may be related to harm from medicines (Pirmohamed et al., 2004) and around 7 per cent of inpatients may suffer harm from medicines, much of which is preventable (Wiffen et al., 2002). A mistake may be considered a relatively minor consequence for the patient. Some, however, result in serious, lasting harm, such as chronic pain, undiagnosed cancers, blindness and even death. In the UK about 10 per cent of inpatient episodes result in errors of some kind, of which about half are preventable (NPSA, 2004a). The Serious Hazards of Transfusion (SHOT) annual report published in 2003 recommended the evaluation of computerised transfusion aids and bar code technology for confirmation that the correct blood is administered. In the period 1996 to 2001, SHOT reported 11 deaths and 60 cases of major morbidity due to incorrect blood component transfused.

Medication errors produce effects from the basis of a sizeable proportion of claims for negligence. The UK medical defence union identify claims directly related to errors in prescribing, monitoring or administering medicines. In addition, incorrect or inappropriate dosage was one of six common reasons for medication errors. Further causes include mental block, blunder because basic arithmetical skills are rusty and confusion about the number of noughts to be shifted in converting between a nanogram, microgram and milligram.

The NPSA (2007) has published seven key actions to improve medication safety:

1. Increase reporting and learning from medication incidents.

2. Implement NPSA safer medication practice recommendations, including the alerts on anticoagulants, injectable medicines and wrong-route errors, published in March 2007.

3. Improve staff skills and competences; health care workers should ensure they have the required work competences and support to use medicines safely.

4. Minimise dosing errors by providing information, training and tools for staff to make calculation of doses easier, and target efforts towards high-risk areas (such as children) and high-risk drugs (such as insulin).

5. Ensure medicines are not omitted.

6. Ensure the correct medicines are given to the correct patients; improve packaging and labelling of medicines and support local

systems that make it harder for staff to select wrong medicines or give medicines to wrong patients.

7. Document patients' medicine allergy status; improve recording of patient allergies, and raise awareness among staff of high-risk products and the importance of knowing the patient's allergy status.

Remove the scope for human error by obviating the need for calculations or simplify any required: base dose on age bands (RCPCH 2004), tables for individual doses showing usual dose range, for infusions tables showing dose rate and flow rate, provision of drugs in an appropriate strength, software to prevent overdoses being prescribed, routine check, check and check!

Further, it has been posited that stringent policies be put into place to prevent errors from occurring. This includes 'No interruption policies' during the prescribing, checking and administration of medicines to patients.

Chapter summary

Without questioning, without having knowledge and skill, the very things we are trying to provide for patients to improve their health and well-being may be the very thing that puts them at risk. Our practice must be cautious and thought through, with integrity and expertise and with a rationale for what we are doing in every step. There is evidence to suggest that knowledge and skill are lacking among qualified practitioners in relation to medication safety and management. However, this can be targeted through sharing good practice, education and monitoring practice. Nurses can make a difference, simply by understanding how to prevent a mistake in the first instance – by not rushing or taking short cuts! Nurses must consider the outcome, not only for the patient but also for themselves as professionals. It is about taking a step back, taking a breath and thinking. Mistakes may happen because we are human, but they do not have to happen because we let them happen.

So what have you learned?

Let's do a quick check. Write down your answers to the following questions or simply tick whether the statement is true or false.

1. Mistakes are a result of poor practice, poor knowledge, inexperience, short cuts and can lead to patient harm.

   True ☐   False ☐

2. List the Five Rights:

   ....

   ....

   ....

   ....

   ....

3. Which age groups are the most vulnerable and at risk?

   0-8 ☐   18-35 ☐   70-100 ☐

4. Name a key NMC document to provide guidance on safe medicine administration.

   ....

5. What is a key resource you can access online or as hard copy to find out about medicine dosages, side effects, indications, etc.

   ....

6. How many tablets would you give to a patient who is prescribed 6.25 mcg of a drug and the stock dose available is 12.5 mcg tablets?

   ....

References and key texts

British National Formulary (2010) *BNF 59*. London: BMA Group and RPS Publishing.

Department of Health (2004) *Building a Safer NHS for Patients: Improving Medication Safety*. London: The Stationery Office.

Dimond, B. (ed.) (2008) *Legal Aspects of Nursing*, 5th edn. London: Pearson.

Kelly, M., Hardwick, K., Moritz, S., Kelner, M., Rickhi, B. and Quan, H. (2005) 'Towards integration: the opinions of health policy makers on complementary and alternative medicine. *Evidence-Based Integrative Medicine* 2 (2): 79–86.

NHSLA (National Health Service Litigation Authority) (2008) *Annual Report*. Available at http://www.nhsla.com/NR/rdonlyres/75CA815D-DF7E-4DB7-90BC-6DCE63A33B24/0/DNVsAnnualReportontheNHSLitigationAuthority Contract200910.pdf.

NMC (Nursing and Midwifery Council) (2004) *Guidelines for the Administration of Medicines*. London: NMC.

NMC (Nursing and Midwifery Council) (2008a) *The Code: Standards of Conduct, Performance and Ethics for Nurses and Midwives*. London: NMC.

NMC (Nursing and Midwifery Council) (2008b) *Standards for Medicines Management*. London: NMC.

NPSA (National Patient Safety Agency) (2004a) *Right Patient–Right Care*. Available at http://www.nrls.npsa.nhs.uk/resources/?entryid45=59805.

NPSA (National Patient Safety Agency) (2004b) *Seven Steps to Patient Safety: An Overview Guide for NHS Staff*. Available at: http://www.npsa.co.uk/patientsafety/improving patient safety/7 steps/.

NPSA (National Patient Safety Agency) (2007) *Safety in Doses: Improving the Use of Medicines in the NHS*. Available at http://npsa.uk/patientsafety/medication-zone/reviews-of-medication-incidents/.

Pirmohamed, M., James, S., Meakin, S., Green, C., Scott, A.K., Walley, T.J., Farrar, K., Park, B.K. and Breckenridge, A.M. (2004) 'Adverse drug reactions as cause of admission to hospital: prospective analysis of 18 820 patients'. *British Medical Journal* 329: 15–19.

RCPCH (The Royal College of Paediatrics and Child Health) (2004) *Safer and Better Medicines for Children*. Available at http://www.rcpch.ac.uk.

SHOT (Serious Hazards of Transfusion Steering Group) (2003) *SHOT Report*. Available at http://www.shotuk.org/shot-reports/reports-and-summaries-2003/.

Wiffen, P., Gill, M., Edwards, J. and Moore, A. (2002) 'Adverse drug reactions in hospital patients: a systematic review of prospective and retrospective studies'. *Bandolier Evidence-Based Healthcare* (Bandolier Extra): 1-15. Available at http://www.ebandolier.com.

Additional reading

Aya, M. (2006) Useful medicines information sources. *Practice Nurse* 32: 32-8.

British Medical Association (2002) *BMA Guide to Drugs and Medicines*. London: Dorling Kindersley.

Chapelhow, C. and Crouch, S. (2007) *Nursing Numeracy: A New Approach*. Cheltenham: Nelson Thornes.

Department of Health (2001) *National Service Framework for Older People*. London: The Stationery Office.

Department of Health (2007) *Saving Lives: Reducing Infection, Delivering Clean and Safe Care*. London: The Stationery Office.

Department of Health (2009) *Better Blood Transfusion Tool Kit: Appropriate Use of Blood*. London: The Stationery Office.

Downie, G., Mackenzie, J. and Williams, A. (2003) *Pharmacology and Medicines Management for Nurses*. Harmondsworth: Penguin.

Eisenhauer, L.A., Hurley, A.C. and Dolan, N. (2007) 'Nurses' reported thinking during medication administration'. *Journal of Nursing Scholarship* 39: 82-7.

Elliott, M. and Liu, Y. (2010) 'The nine rights of medication administration: an overview'. *British Journal of Nursing* 19 (5): 300-5.

Kelly, L.E. and Colby, N. (2003) 'Teaching medication calculations for conceptual understanding'. *Journal of Nursing Education* 42 (10): 431-2.

MHRA (2002) *Adverse Drug Reaction: A Potential Role for Liaison Officers*. London: MHRA.

World Health Organization (1975) *Safety, Efficacy and Utilisation*. Geneva: WHO. Available at http://www.who.int/medicines/areas/quality_safety/safety_efficacy.

Wright, K. (2009) 'Supporting the development of calculating skills in nurses'. *British Journal of Nursing* 18 (7): 399-402.

Websites

http://bnf.org.uk

http://bps.ac.uk

http://www.dh.gov.uk

http://www.mhra.gov.uk

http://www.nhsla.com

http://www.nmc-uk.org

http://www.npsa.uk

http://www.who.int

Chapter 5

Improving knowledge and safety: pharmacological principles

When you have completed this chapter you should:

- have an understanding of essential pharmacological principles
- have an understanding of key drug information: name; indication; therapeutic effect; route, dosage and formulation; side effects; cautions and contra-indications
- understand and apply pharmacological knowledge to promote health and prevent mistakes in medicines management
- be able to apply this knowledge to promote patient education and safety in medicines management

Your starting point

1. Below are different routes of medicine administration. Match the route on the left with the appropriate site of absorption on the right.

   A. Oral   .... Systemic circulation

   B. Sublingual   .... Small intestine

   C. Intramuscular   .... Mucosal membrane

2. Which organ is responsible for metabolism of drugs?

   ....

3. Define 'pharmacology'.

   ....

   ....

4. Match the terms below with the correct meaning.

   A. Pharmacodynamics   .... is the study of therapeutic use and effects of drugs

   B. Pharmacokinetics   .... is what the body does to the drug

   C. Pharmacotherapeutics   .... is what the drug does to the body

5. Which organs are responsible for the excretion of drugs?

   ....

   ....

6. Where are three places where drugs may be stored in your clinical area?

   ....

   ....

   ....

7. How many other names are there for 'morphine sulphate? List at least four.

....

....

....

....

8. Are a side effect and an adverse effect of a drug the same?

Yes ☐   No ☐   Unsure ☐

Introduction

A vital requirement for nurses in safe and effective medicines management is having knowledge of medicines, and in particular of how they work in relation to what they do to the body and what the body does to the drug. Therefore pharmacological principles are key to understanding the patient and their treatment and making safe decisions about this in relation to their medicines.

In an effort to reduce risk and harm and to prevent mistakes, nurses need to be confident of this knowledge and they must be able to share this with patients and indeed learn from patients. A fundamental part of our role is to promote health and prevent illness, and this stems from having sound education and knowledge, and indeed experience.

In Chapter 1 it was identified that a key outcome of nursing practice is safe patient care, where our professional and legal duty of care is not to harm the patient. It also means that we maintain professional standards of care, in promoting health, preventing illness and managing disease. This stems from sharing knowledge and experience, educating our patients and indeed ourselves with regular updates and keeping abreast of changes to clinical practice, research and the recent evidence base upon which these practices are built.

Pharmacological principles

Pharmacology is the study of how drugs affect the function of host tissues or combat infectious organisms (Dale and Haylett, 2004). In most instances a drug's action is to bind selectively to target molecules within the body. Therefore understanding what a drug does and how it works is fundamental.

There are other key terms that you will need to know and understand before we can begin looking at some of the pharmacological issues, to improve your knowledge and understanding of how drugs work and what they do.

Pharmacodynamics is the study of how drugs act and is concerned with what the drug does to the body. It is the effect of the drug at its site of action in the body (Waller et al., 2005). It looks at how drugs modify function of body organs through their effects at the level of individual cells (McLoughlin, 2004).

Pharmacokinetics is what the body does to the drug. It is the effects of the body on drug delivery to its site of action (Waller et al., 2005). It describes the movement of drugs in relation to how the body absorbs, distributes, metabolises and excretes drugs.

Both pharmacokinetics and pharmacodynamics are subject to a number of variables, such as drug-receptor interaction, drug interactions, metabolism and renal elimination.

Patients rely on nursing staff to ensure that their medicines are administered appropriately and safely. It is therefore vital that nurses, midwives and specialist community public health nurses have a sound understanding of the outcome of a drug once it has been administered to a patient.

How do drugs work?

In certain tissues, cells contain receptors and when combined with substances naturally produced in the body, the cells can be stimulated or inhibited. The concept is best explained by analogy to a jigsaw puzzle whereby one piece of the jigsaw, the drug, fits onto another, the receptor, which causes a response. Nearly all drugs will interact with specific components of cells, often found on the cell membrane, and in most cases drugs will bind 'selectively' to target molecules within the body. The response may stimulate naturally occurring stimuli, it may inhibit or block stimuli or it may enhance stimuli. Therefore, drugs acting on sites can be classified and described in terms of their affinity and/or their efficacy.

Affinity = the drug's binding ability

Efficacy = after binding, it is the ability of the drug to affect the receptor and cause a response

The response varies and these are classified accordingly:

- A full agonist binds to the receptor of a cell and triggers a response by that cell, displaying full efficacy at that receptor.

- An agonist stimulates the receptor and produces an effect similar to that of naturally occurring stimuli. Examples of agonists are salbutamol, histamine, noradrenaline, isoprenaline and morphine. How an agonist works can be described by the action of morphine where the effect of the drug mimics the action of natural endorphins at μ-opioid receptors throughout the central nervous system.

- A partial agonist can also bind and activate a given receptor, but it has only partial efficacy at the receptor. Examples of partial agonists include buspirone, aripiprazole, buprenorphine and norclozapine.

- An antagonist occupies the receptor site without producing any effect by preventing the receptor's naturally occurring stimulation. It blocks the action of the agonist. Antagonists have affinity but no efficacy and therefore bind but do not trigger a receptor. Examples include naloxone and atropine. How an antagonist works can be described by the action of atropine where natural acetylcholine is blocked by the atropine molecule and no stimulation occurs.

- An inverse agonist acts on receptors to produce a change opposite to that caused by the agonist (Waller et al., 2005).

With some drugs the action on a receptor may be immediate and direct or the action on the receptor may elicit a chain reaction of events before the final action of the drug is apparent.

Other mechanisms are elicited when substances such as enzymes speed up chemicals in the body – these are enzyme inhibitors. With diuretics, normally salt and water are transported out of the renal tubule back into the body, but if the enzyme action is inhibited this will not occur. The resultant effect is that the diuretic inhibits this action and water and salt are not reabsorbed, pass through the kidney, resulting in diuresis (Trounce, 2000).

Other actions of drugs include: produce replacement for deficient substances; kill bacteria; or cause interference in the movement of naturally occurring ions and prevent nerve or muscle function.

In order to understand what is happening to a drug it is best to think of it in relation to 'its journey through the body'. This journey can be described in four stages:

1. Absorption
2. Distribution
3. Metabolism
4. Elimination.

Absorption

Absorption can be simply explained as the point of interaction. It is the transfer of the drug from the site of administration to the general circulation (Waller et al., 2005).

There are five principles of absorption:

1. Disintegration and dissolution of tablets
2. Passive diffusion
3. Cell membrane and fat solubility of drugs
4. Active transport
5. Pre-systemic metabolism.

At this point it is necessary to explain a few terms. Recall, diffusion is the movement of molecules or particles across a cell membrane. Active transport is the movement of a substance against its concentration energy. In all cells this is usually concerned with accumulating high concentrations of molecules that the cell needs, such as ions, glucose, amino acids. Solubility refers to the ability of compounds to dissolve (remember that fats or lipids are generally not soluble in water – this will be revisited when we discuss metabolism).

The term bioavailability is the ability of a drug to be absorbed and reach the site of action, and this is key in drug absorption. For example, bioavailability is immediate via the intravenous route but takes much longer via the subcutaneous route. Bioavailability can be further explained by comparing the intravenous (IV) route and the oral route. A drug that is administered intravenously has what is referred to as 100 per cent bioavailability as compared to the drug administered orally wherein its bioavailability is significantly less.

This idea will make more sense when we look at various routes of administration and factors influencing absorption of drugs.

First of all, the drug enters the bloodstream, and the time that this takes – the absorption time – is largely dependent upon the route of administration (see Table 5.1). Clearly, this is faster (and indeed more efficient when we think of the drug's bioavailability) if the drug is given intravenously, as it is then introduced directly into systemic circulation.

Table 5.1 **Absorption sites**

Route	Absorption site and time for effect
Oral	Small intestine, 30 minutes
Sublingual	Mucosal membrane, immediate effect
Buccal	Mucosal membrane, immediate effect once absorbed
Subcutaneous	Systemic circulation, slow effect
Intramuscular	Systemic circulation, 15 minutes
Inhalation	Alveoli in lungs, immediate effect but variable in duration of effect
Intravenous	Systemic circulation directly, immediate effect

ACTIVITY 5.1

Can you think of how both oral routes of paracetamol – as an effervescent powder and as a scored tablet – would be absorbed differently and why?

....

....

....

....

....

Drug absorption is dependent on several factors:

- Both chemical and physiological factors influence drug absorption.
- The site of drug administration can alter the rate of drug absorption.
- Drug access to systemic circulation can be limited by the route of administration.

Once absorbed, the drug will produce an effect wherein the drug receptor interaction changes the molecular structure, causing a response. There are a number of factors which can affect the absorption rate and extent to which a drug passes from the gut into circulation. These include acid pH of gastric content, intestinal transit time, gastric emptying time, and drug solubility.

Drug stability may differ where some of the drug is absorbed from the intestine into the blood and some of the absorbed drug is further metabolised by the liver before entering systemic circulation. Therefore the drug may be 'altered' into a different form before it is finally absorbed into systemic circulation. This is called 'first pass effect'. This provides one rationale (of many) for administering drugs via the intravenous route.

Although the oral route of medicine administration is very economical and in most cases is an easy way to administer medicines (whether they be capsules, tablets or a syrup), this route presents the greatest number of barriers to the drug prior to reaching systemic circulation.

Distribution

Following absorption into systemic circulation, drugs permeate organs and tissues. This process is referred to as distribution. This term describes where the drug goes in the body. It is the process by which the drug is transferred reversibly from general circulation into tissues and into blood. For most drugs this occurs by simple diffusion. However, depending on the drug involved, accumulation can occur in different parts of the body. Distribution is affected by several factors.

ACTIVITY 5.2

Can you think of any factors in relation to the patient that may affect distribution?

These factors include:

- Patient body weight
- Clinical condition of the patient
- Drug regimen
- Solubility of the drug.

Additionally, drugs can undergo redistribution from well perfused to poorly perfused tissues.

ACTIVITY 5.3

List those organs that are

Well perfused (have a good blood supply): ....

....

....

Poorly perfused (have a poor blood supply): ....

....

....

This is clinically important when considering the termination of drug action. For example, following intravenous drug administration, a high initial plasma concentration of the drug rapidly enters well perfused tissue. Well perfused organs include the brain, the liver, adrenal glands, kidneys, thyroid, heart, intestines and placenta. Poorly perfused organs include the skin, the skeletal and muscle organs, connective tissue and fat.

Although the distribution of drugs to all organs is relatively straight-forward, more detailed consideration is necessary for two complex systems: the brain, because of the difficulty of drug entry, and the placenta because of the potential for toxicity (Waller et al., 2005). Lipid-soluble, as opposed to water-soluble, drugs readily pass from the blood into tissue, hence the blood–brain barrier. This barrier to water-soluble molecules performs a vital function and is largely owing to reduced capillary permeability (Waller et al., 2005). In addition, lipid-soluble drugs readily cross the placenta; however, maternal circulation predominately controls foetal concentration of a drug. The baby may show effects of a drug given to the mother close to delivery, which may be prolonged because of the reliance on the baby's own immature elimination processes.

Metabolism

Metabolism is the third stage of the drug's journey through the body; however, it may also occur in the final stage, elimination. Because solubility of a drug is a vital property, metabolism is an important process whereby lipid-soluble molecules are converted into water-soluble particles (Waller et al., 2005). The term 'metabolise' means to detoxify, and this is achieved by breaking down a drug into a usable, or soluble, form by liver enzymes, thus making it easier to excrete. Some drugs can modify their own metabolism and that of other drugs by the induction of hepatic enzymes (Dale and Haylett, 2004).

For many drugs, however, there are two phases of drug metabolism. Both of which are complex and require a deep knowledge of chemistry, which is beyond the scope of this book. Suffice here to say that phase one involves three reactions referred to as oxidation, reduction and hydrolysis; and phase two involves conjugation reactions, where the aim is to make the molecule more lipophobic (that is, less lipid soluble) and reduce the possibility of reabsorption in the renal tubules. Drug metabolism can result in the activation or deactivation of the chemical. Enzymes in the liver are responsible for modifying the biochemical composition of drugs and their action is often referred to as xenobiotic metabolism. Most drugs, therefore are 'xenobiotics' or what may be commonly referred to as organic chemicals (Trounce, 2000).

ACTIVITY 5.4

List factors that may affect drug metabolism:

....

....

....

....

....

....

Metabolism occurs mainly in the liver; however, it can also occur in the gut lining, the kidney and the lungs. It is influenced and affected by a variety of factors which include:

- Concurrent drug administration (ingestion of two or more drugs at the same time can affect the rate of metabolism of one or more of the drugs)

- Age
- Liver impairment
- Poor lung function
- Poor renal function
- Whether the patient smokes
- Underlying condition of the patient.

Elimination

Elimination is the removal of a drug from the body. It is often the end point or termination of drug action, in which the drug molecule is expelled in the body's liquid, solid or gaseous waste (Waller et al. 2005). The excretion of a drug and its metabolites occurs in the principal organ of excretion, the kidney. However, some compounds can be excreted in bile or by other routes such as the lungs (Dale and Haylett, 2004).

Renal excretion is a complex process that involves glomerular filtration and active tubular secretion (see Figure 5.1). Within these processes drugs may have properties that allow for active secretion and reabsorption, such as the degree of alkalinity, acidity or lipid solubility. In addition, a drug's half-life may be affected. Glomerular filtration rate (GFR) describes the flow rate of filtered fluid through the kidney and it is the measurement taken. Creatinine clearance rate, which identifies the volume of blood plasma that is cleared of creatinine per unit time, is a useful measure for approximating the GFR. The results of these tests are important in assessing the excretory function of the kidneys. For example, grading of chronic renal insufficiency and dosage of drugs that are primarily excreted via urine are based on GFR (or creatinine clearance).

Half-life can be defined as the amount of time the body takes to eliminate a drug. This reflects the time taken for the plasma drug level to fall to half its initial level. In practice, the half-life reported for a drug is the half-life of the elimination rate measured over the slowest terminal phases of the plasma concentration versus time.

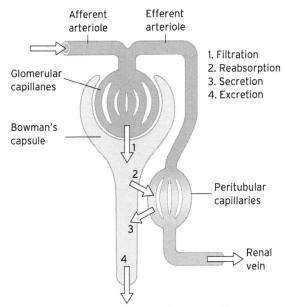

Afferent arteriole
Efferent arteriole

1. Filtration
2. Reabsorption
3. Secretion
4. Excretion

Glomerular capillanes

Bowman's capsule

Peritubular capillaries

Renal vein

Excretion = Filtration − Reabsorption + Secretion

Figure 5.1 **Urinary excretion.**

Example 5.1

After an IV drug is administered, its concentration is halved every hour. Its half-life is 1 hour.

Renal and faecal excretion are the most important routes for elimination. Excretion of drugs varies with age and should be a consideration in drug therapy. If renal impairment is present it may be necessary to reduce drug dosages in order to prevent drug accumulation and further monitor serum creatinine levels closely, to indicate where dosage alterations are needed. This is paramount if renal excretion is an important component of drug elimination.

ACTIVITY 5.5

In your clinical area, obtain the creatinine levels for a patient in your care. What do the figures tell you about this patient's kidney function?

....

....

....

....

Identify the normal creatinine level for an adult: .... mmol/litre

A closer look at drugs

Now that we have looked at what the drug does and indeed what the body does to a drug, let us look at drugs in more detail. Medicines management encapsulates all facets of medicines, and administering medicines safely requires nurses to understand what it is they are giving and why.

Drug nomenclature

ACTIVITY 5.6

List other names for morphine.

....

....

....

....

Nomenclature is the naming of drugs. And the naming can be classified in three ways. Take morphine as an example. Its generic or non-proprietary name is morphine sulphate; its trade names or proprietary names include Sevredol™, Morcap™, MST™; and its chemical name is

$C_{17}H_{19}NO_3 \cdot 5H_2O \cdot SO_4$ – however, this is highly unlikely to be used in clinical practice. Here's why . . .

ACTIVITY 5.7

Can you identify what this drug is?

Endo-a-hydroxymethyl benzeneacetic acid-8-methyl-8-azobicyclo (3-2-1)oct-3-yl ester

Clearly, the chemical name may not be recognised and in clinical practice they are not altogether easily identified. The above, is the chemical name for atropine. Some drugs, however, have many trade names and these may be used instead of a generic name. Some drugs have more obvious names, for example ferrous sulphate, which is also known as Ferron™ and has a commonly recognisable chemical name $FeSO_4$.

However, safety in medicines management requires that the prescription be clear, unambiguous, with drug's names prescribed in their generic or non-proprietary name. All prescriptions should be clearly printed and legible, and abbreviations should be avoided. This is vital in reducing potential error.

ACTIVITY 5.8

Identify the recommendations for prescribers given on the BNF website at http://bnf.org.uk.

Some legal aspects

All drugs are regulated by law that governs their manufacture, supply, storage and use. This was highlighted in Chapter 3, and it is important for nurses to be aware of the legal implications, certainly for controlled drugs while in our use and in patient care. Look again at Table 3.1 to remind yourself of the key legislation in this area.

ACTIVITY 5.9

Where is morphine sulphate stored in your clinical area?

....

....

Refer back to Table 3.1 in Chapter 3. Which legislation governs the storage of morphine sulphate?

....

....

Dosage, formulation and route

What do you know about the medicines you give? What should you know?

ACTIVITY 5.10

List all that you would need to know prior to giving 2-5 mg of morphine sulphate to a patient in severe pain. The medication has been prescribed every 3-4 hours as required, and can be given orally or subcutaneously.

....

....

....

....

....

....

Safe steps in medicine administration has been identified in a previous chapter; however, it is essential, in addition to this, that nurses understand and know the classification and indication for a drug, which entails pharmacological principles and further understanding of what the drug is for and what it will do. In addition, nurses must know the dosage, formulation and route for the drugs they administer and be aware that the dosage and route may vary, altering one or the other.

This is certainly true of morphine and many other drugs. For example, ranitidine can be prescribed as 50 mg intravenously but for an oral dose the recommended dosage is 150 mg (BNF, 2010). Morphine sulphate is available as a modified-release formulation, so, for example, Morcap MR™ would not be the correct formulation to administer where the prescription indicates the drug is to be given 3-4 hourly.

Nurses must be aware of these differences in medicines, their formulations and use.

ACTIVITY 5.11

List all of the known side effects for morphine sulphate.

....

....

....

....

....

....

If your patient develops a respiratory arrest following administration would this be an adverse event? ....

Side effects and adverse events

Side effects are those effects of the drug we are made aware of and therefore we have a responsibility to understand and know prior to administering the medicine to the patient. We must also inform the patient of these. Often we can manage known side effects with other treatments, particularly where the benefit of the drug treatment outweighs the risk of the side effect. Adverse events are not always known and it is important that patients are informed, monitored and assessed during drug therapy, particularly when it is a new drug prescribed.

Safe practice and the prevention of errors

Medicines are drugs which contain chemicals, therefore there is a risk associated with all medicines. How they are used, prescribed, stored and checked should reflect one's knowledge of the drug and safe processes of checking.

Medicines management is not just about the medicine, it is also about patient safety and management of this. The physicality of the medicine and our pharmacological knowledge of what it is and what it does are vitally important to safe practice. How we go about choosing, prescribing, dispensing, educating, obtaining consent, administering, documenting and recording are all important steps. It is a complex process, in which several health care professionals are involved, and it is where the nurse is at the forefront of every stage. In some cases, the nurse is responsible for the patient in all of these stages and the process of safe medicines management.

This brings us to issues of prevention of error. There is a global need to reduce error incidence, ensure patient safety and safe processes in medicines management. Recent NMC regulations regarding skills, for example numeracy, mean that this subject will undoubtedly be an integral part of these learning processes and course development over the coming years.

In previous chapters this has been highlighted, but let's look at issues surrounding dosage calculations and other aspects of calculating in medicine administration where there is the potential for error.

Calculating medication dosages is only one step in the medication administration process, but it has potentially critical outcomes for patients. Errors occur when calculating doses and preparing doses. This is compounded by the two systems used in medicines management: apothecary and metric.

Common measurements for liquid medication, such as a teaspoon (Figure 5.2), are often used as a familiar system of measurement for patients when they are sent home and for those that self-administer.

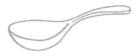

Figure 5.2 A teaspoon should hold 5 ml of liquid but the size of teaspoons can vary so care must be used when measuring a prescribed dose.

However, a teaspoon and the accuracy of the volume can vary and often be more than the prescribed dose.

The unit dose system can eliminate chances of error in drug calculation doses, however it does not totally eradicate it but simply reduces the need for a calculation. This can have a knock-on effect that is detrimental - it would mean less practice with calculations, and lead to the loss of expertise in medication calculation and in turn to error and lack of confidence in calculations. There is sufficient evidence to show that practice is the key to keeping up any skills, and this is certainly true of numeracy and calculation skills in medicines management.

Routes of medicine administration

There are many factors that determine the route of medication administration. The patient/client presentation reveals much about what is prescribed and how it will be given. Rate, accuracy and concentration desired from the drug regimen, patient safety, acceptability and consent, and, most importantly, the patient's/client's condition are all important factors that must be considered.

ACTIVITY 5.12

List all the routes of administration you have experienced in your clinical practice

....

....

....

....

....

There are many ways in which medicines can be delivered to the patient in order to achieve a therapeutic effect, treat, cure or manage their care. For each route there is required knowledge and skill to safely administer and monitor the effect.

Drugs can be given orally, sublingually, buccally, intravenously, by injection (intramuscularly, intradermally, subcutaneously), rectally, vaginally, by inhalation, topically, aurally, and into the eye or nose. There are also many routes that only skilled practitioners may use to administer medicines: intra-arterially, intra-articularly, and via an epidural.

Oral route

The oral route of administration is the most common, most economical and most practical. However, it is not always a route that can be used.

ACTIVITY 5.13

What would prevent the oral route from being prescribed?

....

....

....

....

....

....

Oral preparations come in a variety of forms and formulations: tablets or capsules, a chewable or scored tablet; an effervescent or dispersible formulation; tablets that are film, enteric or sugar coated or of a modified-released formulation for long-acting or sustained release; liquids such as linctus, syrup or suspension; and lozenges. Some of these forms indicate how a drug works or where they are absorbed in the body.

For example, enteric-coated (e/c) preparations are surrounded by a coating which does not dissolve until it reaches more alkaline conditions of the duodenum, so that stomach acid is protected from unwanted effects of the drug (John and Stevenson, 2005). Modified-release (MR) or slow/sustained release (SR) formulations release the drug over time, and if in capsule form these capsules must not be tampered with, opened or altered as this could affect the release time and desired effect of the drug (BNF, 2010).

It is important for nurses always to seek advice or to refer to manufacturer guidelines on how to administer formulations safely. Associated factors that can also affect the drug action include water temperature, acidic juices, or indigestion remedies taken with orally prescribed drugs. Instructions such as 'take on an empty stomach' or 'take 1 hour after eating' are significant. The presence or absence of food in the stomach can affect the rate of absorption and the amount of the drug absorbed, such as flucloxacillin, or gastric irritation may result for some drugs taken on an empty stomach, such as aspirin (BNF, 2010).

Sublingual and buccal routes

Other routes of administration that are not particularly popular but are important to understand are the sublingual (S/L) and buccal route. The sublingual drug is placed under the tongue, providing a faster onset of action and avoiding inactivation by the liver before reaching systemic circulation (Goodman et al., 1992). However, if this preparation is swallowed the drug may have no effect. The buccal route requires the drug to be placed within the pouch of the inner gum and cheek. Both routes are susceptible to inefficiency if the patient's mouth is dry or if the drug is not positioned correctly.

Subcutaneous route

Injections require additional training and understanding of the skill required to administer the drug safely and with as little discomfort to the patient as possible. Drugs given via the subcutaneous route are delivered into fatty or subcutaneous tissue, just below the outer layers of skin. The needle is injected beneath the epidermis into the fat and connective tissue underlying the dermis (Endacott et al., 2009). There is still debate about the angle of injection for this route and delivery is dependent upon the needle size. Common drugs given this way are insulin and heparins, which would be broken down if given

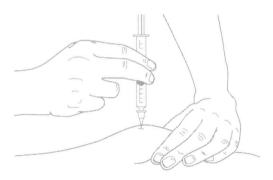

Figure 5.3 Subcutaneous injection technique.

orally due to digestive enzymes in the saliva (BNF, 2010). Today it is more common to see the drugs in 'pens' or as 'pre-loaded' syringes. The small-size needle permits insertion at 90 degrees (Figure 5.3). However, if a needle is placed on a syringe, it is recommended to use a 4-8 mm needle and to inject at 90 degrees, and that anything greater is injected at 45 degrees (Workman, 1999; Greenway, 2004; Endacott et al., 2009).

The condition of the patient must be a consideration and assessment of the sites ongoing. There are various sites for this injection route: the upper outer aspect of the humerus, the upper anterior surface of the thighs, or the abdominal area proximal to the naval (Figure 5.4). Some drugs are licensed to be administered in designated sites or in a specified way. For example, Celexane™, a low molecular weight heparin that is given to prevent deep vein thrombosis (DVT), must be given in the abdomen and not in the arm. If patients self-administer, then the abdomen is often a preferred site and has been reported as less painful than other sites. Patients may find, however, that it is easier to self-inject into their upper thigh.

Practitioners must assess the subcutaneous site and ideally inject into a fold of skin. Drugs administered to the subcutaneous site do not have an immediate effect and only small volumes can be given this way (up to 2 ml is acceptable) (Workman, 1999; Endacott et al., 2009). For some treatments, larger volumes are given, for example diamorphine pumps in palliative care. In such cases, however, absorption may be unpredictable (John and Stevenson, 2005). Often the onset of action

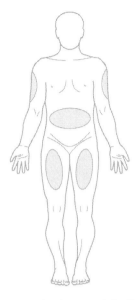

Figure 5.4 Injection sites for subcutaneous injections.

with the subcutaneous route is delayed or slow owing to the very nature of the fatty tissue and lack of blood supply.

Intramuscular route

The intramuscular route of administration is used less today largely because of technological advances in, for example, pain control, where a continuous infusion or what is often called 'patient controlled analgesia' (PCA) or analgesia given via an epidural infusion may be best indicated. Intramuscular (IM) injections are indicated for anti-emetic treatment, some forms of pain relief, immunisations, steroid and fertility treatments and for some anti-psychotropic medicines. The onset of action for this route is quicker as the drug reaches systemic circulation faster. However, there is added risk to the patient and to the practitioner.

Common sites for intramuscular injections include:

● The deltoid muscle (Figure 5.5c) up to 1 ml (Workman, 1999; Greenway, 2004; Endacott et al., 2009).

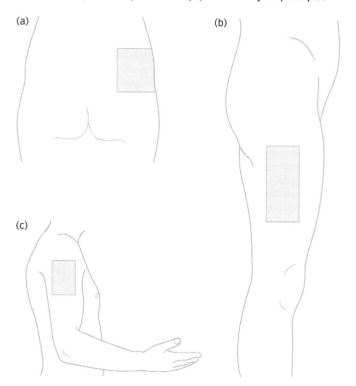

Figure 5.5 Injection sites (a) gluteal, (b) quadriceps and (c) deltoid.

- The rectus formalis and vastus lateralis muscles of the thigh (Figure 5.5b) up to 5 ml (in adults) and 4 ml in children (Greenway, 2004; Endacott et al., 2009).
- The dorsogluteal and ventrogluteal muscles of the buttock (Figure 5.5a) up to 4 ml (Greenway, 2004).

For each of these sites there is a limitation on the volume that can be injected safely and individual patient assessment is necessary. The appropriate site must be assessed and it is vital that nurses are aware of key considerations: the drug, the volume and, more importantly, the patient.

Assessment of the patient should include their age, weight and muscle mass, and understanding key anatomical features is necessary in order to safely identify and 'landmark' the site for injection (see Table 5.2 and Figures 5.6 and 5.7).

Table 5.2 How to landmark injection sites

Anatomical site	Landmarking instructions
Deltoid	To locate, identify the acromial process of the humerus and the point of the arm in line with the axilla, insert 2.5 cm below the acromium process (see Figure 5.6)
Rectus formalis and vastus lateralis	To locate, measure a hand's breadth laterally down from the greater trochanter and a hand's breadth from the knee. Identify the middle third of the muscle and insert
Dorsogluteal	To locate, draw an imaginary line horizontally across from the top of the buttock cleft to the greater trochanter of the femur. Draw a second line vertically midway along the first line, inject in the 'upper outer quadrant of the upper outer quadrant'
Ventrogluteal (*recommended deep IM injection site)	To locate, place palm of your right hand on the greater trochanter of patient's left hip (or left hand onto right hip) – see Figure 5.7 Extend incisor finger to touch the anterior superior iliac crest Stretch middle finger to form a 'V' as far as possible along the iliac crest Insert in the middle of the 'V'

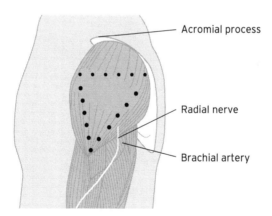

Acromial process

Radial nerve

Brachial artery

Figure 5.6 The location of the deltoid muscle for injection.

Intravenous route

The intravenous route carries with it the greatest risk of all routes, with the exception of epidural, for which specialist training is required (most nursing practitioners are not skilled or qualified to insert these devices). Administration directly into systemic circulation has an

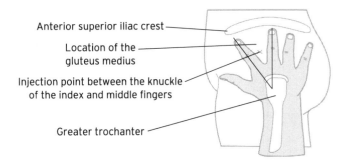

Anterior superior iliac crest

Location of the gluteus medius

Injection point between the knuckle of the index and middle fingers

Greater trochanter

Figure 5.7 **How to landmark the ventrogluteal injection site.**

immediate effect, and hence, an immediate adverse effect. There is an associated risk for anaphylaxis due to the unpredictability and rapid effect of IV injection (RCN, 2010). For this reason, it can also be the most hazardous route.

There is a great deal of information that you must know and understand prior to administering a drug intravenously, for example drug concentration, rate of administration, compatibility, accepted device and equipment for administration.

Example 5.2

A drug given too fast or mixed incorrectly can have devastating consequences. For example, if furosemide is given too fast (greater than 4 mg/min) this could result in transient deafness; if vancomycin is administered too fast (greater than 10 mg per min) then hypotension, shock and cardiac arrest may result (GSTT, 2009; BNF, 2010).

Manufacturer instructions stipulate the final concentration when mixing and preparing IV drugs, and administration rates that must be adhered to. Drugs administered via the intravenous route should be administered via an infusion device and with the appropriate equipment for that device. It is the nurse's responsibility to know, understand and undergo instruction and training on how to use these devices in practice.

The intravenous route should only be used when no other route is available (BMA, 1993; RCN, 2010). The decision for this route must be dependent upon key considerations:

- Patient's general health
- Severity of the patient's condition (Scales, 2008)
- Urgency of the medicinal effect required (Scales, 2008)
- Part of the body to be treated (Scales, 2008).

Vascular access devices

There are different types of devices used to administer medicines intravenously. Collectively they may be referred to as vascular access devices (VADs) and can be categorised in three ways:

- Peripheral venous access devices (PVADs)
- Midline catheter (MC)
- Central venous access devices (CVADs).

Device selection should reflect the needs of the patient, the indicated treatment and duration of therapy or treatment.

Practice guidelines

Choosing the correct device (PVADs):

- The smallest gauge and shortest length should be selected for the prescribed therapy (RCN, 2005).
- 14 gauge for rapid administration of fluids and blood (Scales, 2008); emergency; trauma; haemorrhage.
- 20 gauge or 22 gauge for hydration fluids and antibiotics are less likely to cause mechanical phlebitis (Scales, 2008) and less likely to obstruct blood flow within the vein (Tagalakis et al., 2002).

Insertion of the device (PVADs):

- Non-sterile gloves should be worn (RCN, 2005).
- 2 per cent chlorhexidine in 70 per cent isopropyl alcohol recommended for skin cleansing prior to insertion (RCN, 2005; Pratt et al., 2007).
- Once the skin has been cleansed, it should not be re-palpated (RCN, 2005).

Sites should aim to be in the peripheral extremities of the arm, ideally the cephalic vein (see Figures 5.8 and 5.9).

1 Digital dorsal veins
2 Dorsal metacarpal veins
3 Dorsal venous network
4 Cephalic vein
5 Basilic vein

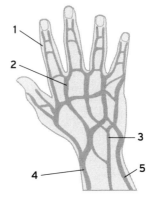

Figure 5.8 The veins of the hand.

1 Cephalic vein
2 Median cubital vein
3 Accessory cephalic vein
4 Basilic vein
5 Cephalic vein
6 Median antebrachial vein

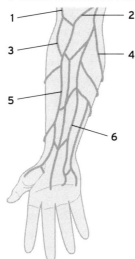

Figure 5.9 The veins of the forearm.

Peripheral devices

Peripheral devices (PVADs) are indicated for short-term use and should therefore be changed every 72 hours or sooner if there are signs of phlebitis (Scales, 2008). However, there are recommendations that indicate the timeframe should be 72-96 hours (Department of Health, 2007) or sooner if there is evidence of phlebitis or infiltration (RCN, 2010).

There are numerous complications that can arise from these devices, including: bruising, local infection, septicaemia, phlebitis, thrombophlebitis, infiltration and/or extravasation, and anaphylaxis. Therefore it is imperative that nurses know the symptoms and recognise these early on in order to prevent their worsening. Key considerations start with the patient, effective communication, education and proactive assessment and routine monitoring.

ACTIVITY 5.14

For each of the complications listed below, write down at least three signs and symptoms:

Local infection: ....

....

Phlebitis: ....

....

Infiltration: ....

....

Extravasation: ....

....

Infection is caused by contamination, which can occur at any stage during infusion therapy – cannula insertion, changing giving sets, medication and fluid administration, inspecting the site, dressing application and changes – or if the device is in situ for longer than the recommended time. Therefore, prevention at all stages is essential, which includes a non-touch technique and hand washing before and after patient interaction (Pratt, 2005).

Good assessment and frequent monitoring are fundamental, and practitioners must have the requisite knowledge when selecting the appropriate size and type of device indicated for the patient. In addition, the practitioner should have appropriate dressing education and training; knowledge of the medicines and fluids administered; and skills in documentation and reporting.

Phlebitis means inflammation of the vein and it can be classified as either chemical, physical or mechanical.

Often the cause is from the type of medicine or fluid administered, where a vesicant or irritable substance such as antibiotics, strong sodium or potassium chloride has irritated the vein wall. Further consideration of the infusion time and dilution, the site and condition of the veins can help to minimise the occurrence of phlebitis. It is essential to consider the patient's condition and ensure that the device is appropriate in size and type. Prevention necessitates ongoing assessment and frequent monitoring where early recognition of the signs and symptoms of phlebitis can deter this complication. Nurses must be vigilant and at the first signs of phlebitis they need to document and report findings and continue to monitor the site and patient response to therapy.

Infiltration is very different from an infection and can be caused by damage to the catheter itself or by fibrin sheath formation. Migration and dislodgement of the device or partial or total displacement of the cannulae may also be the cause. Consideration of the patient, particularly those with fragile veins or poor venous access, needs to be a priority. Other causes of infiltration include: poor technique at cannulation; incorrect method of administration of fluids and medicines; lack of monitoring the infusion; poor assessment of site; and not recognising symptoms of infiltration.

Again, prevention is key, and this requires practitioners to vigilantly assess and recognise early symptoms of infiltration during infusion therapy. Intravenous infusions must be closely monitored and assessed – this includes listening to patients particularly when the infusion is reported as 'troublesome' or 'positional'. Early signs often indicate that there is a problem – when the dressing is wet or leakage at the site is noted. This is quickly followed by swelling and reported pain. Often palpation of the site is painful, cold and blanching can occur. This is clearly very different from an infection and can worsen and lead to cellulitus if not managed appropriately at the first instance of infiltration. Patients will require gentle handling and it can take days or weeks for the condition to improve, or worsen. It is imperative that nurses have the required knowledge and skill to recognise infiltration and that they report and document findings and include patients in education and prevention.

Extravasation is a serious complication and the incidence can lead to devastating consequences for the patient, leaving them with disfigurement or disability and a case for litigation. The cause is similar to that of infiltration where it may be the catheter itself that is damaged or there is fibrin sheath formation. Dislodgement of the device, partial or total displacement of the cannulae and fragile veins or poor venous access are also potential causes. Knowledge deficit reflected in poor technique at cannulation or incorrect methods of administration of vesicant fluids are key causative factors.

A vesicant fluid is one which can cause irritation to the vein. Some examples include: potassium chloride (>40 mmol), sodium bicarbonate (>5 per cent), calcium chloride and other drugs such as gluconate, aciclovir, amphotericin, digoxin, diazepam, dextrose 5 per cent, cefotaxin, mannitol, and cytotoxic drugs.

A vitally important safety element when administering these types of fluids is patient monitoring. A lack of monitoring of the infusion and the site can contribute to extravasation. This is further contributed by poor assessment and not recognising the symptoms which are different from infiltration. In extravasation the patient may report burning, stinging or pain at the site. This is often accompanied with redness, followed by blistering and ulceration and necrosis of the tissue.

Patients at greater risk of extravasation include:

- Those with small fragile veins or thrombosed veins
- Those with chronic disease, cancer, peripheral vascular disease, diabetes
- Those with impaired circulation or who suffer from obesity
- Confused or sedated patients, or those who are unable to speak or have a language barrier
- Those who have undergone multiple cannulation/venepuncture.

Extravasation is a well recognised complication of chemotherapy (Hyde and Dougherty, 2008) but it is generally under-diagnosed, underreported and underrated. The reported incident rate is low but has been higher in peripheral devices. This complication can result with central devices and has occurred in implanted devices, but often detection is delayed and therefore the severity of the complication is greater.

It is vital that practitioners working with chemotherapy and cytotoxic drug therapy have sound knowledge about these drugs and the potential damage that can arise. Extravasation can result in severe damage, depending on the site and the amount and concentration of the drug. Ulceration can develop over a period of days or weeks and the outcome may be grim for those patients who will require plastic surgery or who face the possibility of disability or loss of function.

The complications that can arise with peripheral devices are summarised in Table 5.3.

Table 5.3 Complications associated with peripheral devices

Complication	Clinical signs and symptoms
Infection	Localised redness, heat, swelling and pain, may have fever; can lead to systemic infection (pyrexia, positive blood cultures, rigors, elevated ESR)
Phlebitis	Red 'tracking' from the vein site along the path of the cannula; pain; tenderness; erythema; can lead to infective phlebitis and cause long-term damage to the vein
Infiltration	Localised oedema and swelling; cold or coolness at the site, blanching of the site, leakage at the site; change in infusion flow; pain; can lead to cellulitis and limb dysfunction
Extravasation	Burning, stinging or pain and redness at the site, followed by blistering, then ulceration and necrosis of the surrounding tissue and in some serious cases can result in full thickness skin loss and muscle and tendon necrosis; can lead to permanent scarring, amputation and disability

Midline and central venous access devices

Midline and central venous access devices (CVADs) have an altogether different indication from peripheral devices and are often required for longer treatment and care and for the acutely ill patient. It is vital that nurses undertake additional training and competence assessment in order to manage and care for these devices safely.

Midline catheters are the longer in length (7.5-20 cm) and are inserted just above or below the antecubital fossa. Their placement into the large vein of the upper arm provides good blood flow and decreases the risk of chemical phlebitis and disperses drugs rapidly. Their duration is for up to 4 weeks; however, they must be inserted under aseptic and sterile conditions by a highly skilled and specially trained nurse or a medical officer. There are fewer associated complications with midline catheters in comparison to CVADs.

A *central venous access device* (CVAD) is any vascular access device that terminates in a central vein. There are several types of these devices:

- Non-tunnelled
- Tunnelled
- Peripherally inserted central catheters (PICCs)
- Implantable ports.

Their indication differs from that for peripheral venous access devices (PVADs) (see Table 5.4). One advantage is that the delivery of drugs and fluids is direct into fast-flowing central circulation which therefore decreases the risk of chemical phlebitis and ensures rapid distribution and immediate clinical effect.

Complications associated with CVADs are similar to those for PVADs but can be much more severe and in many cases they can be life threatening (Scales, 2010). They include:

Table 5.4 **CVAD indication (adapted from Scales, 2010)**

Short-term use (<7 days)	Intermediate use (1–4 weeks)	Long-term use (1 month – 1 year)	Long-term use (>1 year)
Peripheral catheter (PC)	MC if irritant infusates	PICC	Tunnelled CVAD
● non-irritant infusates			
● change every 72 hours (Department of Health, 2007)	PICC if irritant infusates	Tunnelled CVAD	Implantable port
Non-tunnelled CVAD		Implantable port	
● irritant infusates or if PC access not available			

- Cardiac arrhythmia
- Extravasation
- Infection
- Anaphylaxis
- Pneumothorax
- Air embolism
- Thrombosis
- Haemorrhage.

ACTIVITY 5.15

For each of the complications listed below, write down at least three signs and symptoms.

Pneumothorax: ....

....

Infection: ....

....

Air embolism: ....

....

Reactions and sensitivities can result at any time during intravenous therapy, regardless of the device or the drug. Penicillins are strongly linked to anaphylaxis and can be a trigger for this allergic response and there is always a risk if the patient has not had the drug before (Downie et al., 2003). Reactions can be mild to severe and can result in anaphylactic shock and death.

ACTIVITY 5.16

Access the website of the Resuscitation Council at www.resus.org.uk and review the treatment guidelines for anaphylaxis and algorithms.

With any drug route, practitioners should consider the effect that the drug will have and the onset of action and where this occurs.

Rectal route

The rectal route is effective but not always acceptable due to cultural differences and patient choice and dignity. When other routes are not options, however – if, for example, the patient is vomiting, unconscious or sedated – this is an effective route for systemic pain control or anti-emetic administration as a suppository. Compared with the oral route, there is less immediate breakdown by the liver, although absorption is generally slower. Patients should be lying on their side with one leg raised. Privacy and dignity is of the utmost concern and nurses need to be aware of the use of lubricant, gloves and safe handling of the patient.

Inhalation route

The inhalation route is very common and is an effective way to deliver drugs or self-administer to all ages of patients/clients. It can provide a local effect or a systemic effect. An important consideration for drugs delivered in this way is technique. Even with excellent technique, only 10 per cent of the dose reaches the lungs (Brown, 2004). Therefore patient/client education and staff education is paramount to deliver the drug effectively, with the correct air flow and using optimum equipment for the patient/client needs.

Topical route

And, finally, the topical route, which is probably the most popular, considering the large number of medications that can be given this way, with or without a prescription. This method of administration provides a local effect or a systemic effect. As with other routes, there are special considerations, for example application onto a broken skin surface must be avoided in order for the drug to pass into systemic circulation. The drug is released slowly, the rate depending on what the topical drug is and how it is administered. Special instructions and manufacturer guidelines must be followed, for example avoiding contact with eyes and washing hands immediately after application if it is a cream, or changing the site if it is a patch.

Eye drops

Eye drops and other ophthalmologic drugs vary in how they are given and where the drop or ointment is delivered. It is imperative that the nurse is knowledgeable and understands the desired effect of the drug indicated. For some ophthalmologic drugs, drops directly onto the pupil may be indicated to cause pupillary reaction here; for others the drops should be instilled into the lower fornix of the eye, and it is imperative that the tip of the dropper does not touch the patient's eyelid.

Ear drops

Ear drops require additional knowledge and skill, and the age of the patient is a key consideration. Ideally the patient is supine with the affected ear upright, and on an adult the pinna of the ear should be held to straighten the ear canal. Drops should be administered without the dropper touching the ear. Patients should be encouraged to lie on their side and wait 3-5 minutes.

Chapter summary

This chapter has provided more detail about medicines and has addressed pharmacological principles that practitioners must be aware of and understand in order to administer medicines safely. There are a multitude of routes and methods, and these have been highlighted, with a clear message that for each there is specific knowledge and skill needed.

For any route of administration, knowledge is key - of what the drug is and what it will do, how it will work and the outcome of its desired effect. Patients need to be informed and practitioners need to have knowledge and skill. In all administration of medicines, local policies and guidelines for safe practice must be followed. Hand washing and a non-touch technique are essential in handling medicines and between direct patient care.

Medicines need to be understood and safe practice needs to reflect this knowledge.

So what have you learned?

Let's do a quick check. Write down your answers to the following questions or simply tick whether the statement is true or false.

1. Pharmacotherapeutics is the study of the therapeutic use and effects of drugs.

   True ☐   False ☐

2. Affinity is a term to describe a drug's binding ability.

   True ☐   False ☐

3. List the four stags of a drug's journey through the body.

   ....

   ....

   ....

   ....

4. Give an example of an agonist.

   ....

5. Give an example of an antagonist.

   ....

6. Three routes of administration are listed. Match the columns to indicate how long it takes for an effect.

   A. Oral route   ....   15-20 minutes
   B. Intravenous route   ....   30-40 minutes
   C. Intramuscular route   ....   Immediate effect

7. Of all the routes of drug administration, which carries with it the greatest risk to the patient?

   ....

8. List four potential complications of intravenous infusion therapy.

....

....

....

....

References and key texts

BNF (British National Formulary) (2010) *BNF 59*. London: BMA Group and RPS Publishing.

Brown, R. (2004) 'Drug delivery systems 2: pulmonary and parental formulations'. *Airways Journal* 2 (1): 43-6.

Dale, M.M. and Haylett, D.G. (2004) *Pharmacology Condensed*. Edinburgh: Churchill Livingstone.

Department of Health (2007) *Saving Lives: Reducing Infection, Delivering Clean and Safe Care*. London: The Stationery Office.

Downie, G., Mackenzie, J. and Williams, A. (2003) *Phamacology and Medicines Management for Nurses*, 3rd edn. Edinburgh: Churchill Livingstone.

Endacott, R., Jevon, P. and Cooper, S. (2009) *Clinical Nursing Skills: Core and Advanced*. Oxford: Oxford University Press.

Galbraith, A., Bullock, S., Manias, E., Hunt, B. and Richards, A. (2007) *Fundamentals of Pharmacology: An Applied Approach for Nursing and Health*. Harlow: Pearson.

Goodman, L.S., Gilman, A., Goodman-Gilman, A. and Rall, T.W. (1992) *Goodman and Gilman's The Pharmalogical Basis of Therapeutics*. Vol 2. New York: Macmillan.

Greenway, K. (2004) 'Using the ventrogluteal site for intramuscular injections'. *Nursing Standard* 18 (25): 39-42.

GSTT (Guy's and St Thomas' NHS Foundation Trust) (2009) *General Guidance on Administration of Intravenous Therapy*. London: GSTT.

Hyde, L. and Dougherty, L. (2008) 'Safe handling of cytotoxic drugs'. In L. Dougherty and S. Lister (eds), *The Royal Marsden Hospital Manual of Clinical Nursing Procedures*, 7th edn. Oxford: Blackwell.

McLoughlin, C. (2004) 'Diuretic drugs'. *Professional Nurse* 20 (2): 50-1.

Pratt, R.J. (2005) *Preventing Healthcare-associated Infections: An Essential Component of Patient Safety*. Available at http://www.saferhealthcare.org.uk/HI/InfectionControl/WhatWeKnow.

Pratt, R.J., Pellowe, C.M., Wilson, J.A. et al. (2007) *Epic 2: National Evidence-based Guidelines for Preventing Healthcare-associated Infections in NHS Hospitals in England*. Available at http://www.rcn.org.uk.

RCN (Royal College of Nursing) (2005) *Standards for Infusion Therapy*. London: RCN.

RCN (Royal College of Nursing) (2010) *Standards for Infusion Therapy*, 2nd edn. London: RCN.

Scales, K. (2008) 'Intravenous therapy: a guide to good practice'. *British Journal of Nursing* (IV Therapy Suppl.) 17(1a): S4-12.

Scales, K. (2010) 'Central venous access devices: Part 2 For intermediate and long-term use'. *British Journal of Nursing* 19 (5): S20-5.

Tagalakis, V., Kahn, S.R., Libman, M. and Blostein, M. (2002) 'The epidemiology of peripheral vein infusion thrombophlebitis: a critical review'. *The American Journal of Medicine* 113: 146-51.

Trounce, J. (2000) *Clinical Pharmacology for Nurses*, 16th edn. Edinburgh: Churchill Livingstone.

Waller, D.G., Renwick, A.G. and Hillier, K. (2005) *Medical Pharmacology and Therapeutics*. 2nd edn. Edinburgh: Elsevier Saunders.

Workman, B. (1999) 'Safe injection techniques'. *Nursing Standard* 13 (39): 47-53.

Additional reading

Copping, C. (2005) 'Preventing and reporting drug administration errors'. *Nursing Times* 101: 32.

Department of Health (2008) *Clean, Safe Care: Reducing Infections and Saving Lives*. London: The Stationery Office.

Dougherty, L. (2008) 'IV therapy: recognising the differences between infiltration and extravasation'. *British Journal of Nursing* 17 (14): 896-901.

Dougherty, L. and Lamb, J. (eds) (2008) *Intravenous Therapy in Nursing Practice*. Oxford: Blackwell.

Greenstein, B. and Gould, D. (2004) *Trounce's Clinical Pharmacology for Nurses*. Edinburgh: Churchill Livingstone.

Jordan, S., Griffith, H. and Griffith, R. (2003) 'Administration of medicines. Part 2: Pharmacology'. *Nursing Standard* 18: 345.

King, R.L. (2004) 'Nurses' perception of their pharmacology knowledge'. *Journal of Advanced Nursing* 45: 393-400.

MHRA (2002) *Report on the Safety of Herbal Medicinal Products*. London: MHRA.

Rang, H.P., Dale, M.M., Ritter, J.M. and Moore, P.K. (2003) *Pharmacology*, 5th edn. Edinburgh: Churchill Livingstone.

Wiffen, P., Mitchell, M., Shelling, M. and Stoner, N. (2007) *Oxford Handbook of Clinical Pharmacy*. Oxford: Oxford University Press.

Wright, S. (2002) 'Swallowing difficulties protocol: medication administration'. *Nursing Standard* 17 (14/15): 43-5.

Zayback, A., Gumes, U.Y., Tamsel, L. and Eser, I. (2007) 'Does obesity prevent the needle from reaching muscle in intramuscular injections?' *Journal of Advanced Nursing* 58: 552-6.

Websites

http://www.bjs.co.uk

http://bnf.org.uk

http://bps.ac.uk

http://www.resus.org.uk

http://www.rcn.org.uk

Pratt, R.J. (2005) *Preventing Healthcare-associated Infections: An Essential Component of Patient Safety*. Available at http://www.saferhealthcare. org.uk/HI/InfectionControl/WhatWeKnow.

Pratt, R.J., Pellowe, C.M., Wilson, J.A. et al. (2007) *Epic 2: National Evidence-based Guidelines for Preventing Healthcare-associated Infections in NHS Hospitals in England*. Available at http://www.rcn.org.uk.

RCN (Royal College of Nursing) (2005) *Standards for Infusion Therapy*. London: RCN.

RCN (Royal College of Nursing) (2010) *Standards for Infusion Therapy*, 2nd edn. London: RCN.

Scales, K. (2008) 'Intravenous therapy: a guide to good practice'. *British Journal of Nursing* (IV Therapy Suppl.) 17 (19): S4-12.

Scales, K. (2010) 'Central venous access devices: Part 2 For intermediate and long-term use'. *British Journal of Nursing* 19 (5): S20-5.

Tagalakis, V., Kahn, S.R., Libman, M. and Blostein, M. (2002) 'The epidemiology of peripheral vein infusion thrombophlebitis: a critical review'. *The American Journal of Medicine* 113: 146-51.

Trounce, J. (2000) *Clinical Pharmacology for Nurses*, 16th edn. Edinburgh: Churchill Livingstone.

Waller, D.G., Renwick, A.G. and Hillier, K. (2005) *Medical Pharmacology and Therapeutics*. 2nd edn. Edinburgh: Elsevier Saunders.

Workman, B. (1999) 'Safe injection techniques'. *Nursing Standard* 13 (39): 47-53.

Additional reading

Copping, C. (2005) 'Preventing and reporting drug administration errors'. *Nursing Times* 101: 32.

Department of Health (2008) *Clean, Safe Care: Reducing Infections and Saving Lives*. London: The Stationery Office.

Dougherty, L. (2008) 'IV therapy: recognising the differences between infiltration and extravasation'. *British Journal of Nursing* 17 (14): 896-901.

Dougherty, L. and Lamb, J. (eds) (2008) *Intravenous Therapy in Nursing Practice*. Oxford: Blackwell.

Greenstein, B. and Gould, D. (2004) *Trounce's Clinical Pharmacology for Nurses*. Edinburgh: Churchill Livingstone.

Chapter 6

Clinical decision making

When you have completed this chapter you should:

- have an understanding of key skills in clinical decision making
- be able to review essential issues in medicines management such as patient consent, drug concordance, refusal of treatment, infection control
- understand and be able to apply effective communication skills to manage patients and their medicines safely and effectively
- be able to apply this knowledge to promote patient safety in medicines management

Your starting point

1. Identify three sources of evidence used in clinical practice, when administering medicines.

   ....

   ....

   ....

2. Can you list any contributing factors to a medication error wherein the patient received the incorrect drug?

   ....

   ....

   ....

3. What do you think are key considerations when obtaining consent from a patient when administering their medicine?

   ....

   ....

   ....

4. Do you agree with putting medicine in a patient's food so that they will take it?

   Yes ☐   No ☐   Unsure ☐

5. Is medicine administration considered a non-touch technique?

   Yes ☐   No ☐   Unsure ☐

Introduction

It is essential that nurses are confident in their clinical decision making and communication skills, as these are fundamental to the outcomes of medicines management. Nurses need to be able to make decisions about patient care and use sound clinical judgement. In order to do this, nurses must have knowledge of evidence and rationale for their actions and an understanding of the patients and their needs. Communicating effectively requires understanding the situation, developing a question in order to solve the problem. Thus a systematic approach, as identified in other aspects of medicines management, is key.

In order to practise safely within medicines management it is important that nurses have knowledge of a range of sources and evidence that will help to inform clinical decision making (Lawson and Hennefer, 2010) and have an understanding of legislation and specific statutory instruments that are in place to protect patients. Our professional role and duty of care requires that we advocate for patients in our care and ensure safe and effective standards of practice and care. Therefore, it is important to reflect on your role and how this will impact upon the decisions that you make for your patients, other members of the inter-professional team and with regard to safe practice outcomes. A fundamental skill for practitioners is to effectively communicate and engage with patients and the team, particularly when faced with challenging situations.

Knowledge is the first step to safe practice and essential when clinical decision making is needed.

Evidence-based practice

The NMC (2008a) indicates that nurses must justify their actions and their omissions. This requires an understanding of what it is we do and why. A significant catalyst to one's actions comes from the rationale for what we do. This is highly influenced by evidence and indeed research that purposes to support our decision making and provide those reasons that help in our understanding for the decisions we make.

ACTIVITY 6.1

Have you read an article or government paper recently that influenced your practice? What was the impact, if any, on your practice?

....

....

....

....

....

....

Evidence in medicines management comes from a variety of sources. The most likely resource is the British National Formulary (BNF) which we have referred to in previous chapters and with which you should now be comfortable. In addition there are strategies and guidance from a variety of organisations, with the NMC being the most influential and providing key standards for practice. Further, the Department of Health and other government bodies, which were reviewed in Chapter 3, highlight how influential research is to our ever-changing practice and that learning from mistakes is a fundamental part of change. These initiatives have played a significant part in shaping practice though evidence and shared knowledge.

Evidence-based practice is a means of sharing best practice and evidence that shapes service delivery and excellence in patient care. It is essential that the health service can demonstrate excellence and quality standards and control. Treatment strategies are influenced by research and evidence which help to develop practice frameworks, protocols and guidelines.

Therefore, strength in clinical decision making is underpinned by one's understanding and application of evidence-based practice guidelines and supporting research.

ACTIVITY 6.2

Identify one practice protocol or guideline used in your clinical area that has recently been influenced and changed as a result of research.

....

....

In addition, legislation and expert opinion can also have an impact on our actions and indeed our decision making.

The Mental Capacity Act 2010

Let us first review an important piece of legislation that has a significant impact on decision making: the Mental Capacity Act 2010.

ACTIVITY 6.3

Access the Mental Capacity Act 2010 from the web link www.opsi.gov.uk.

Key sections of the Act are:

s 1(2) A person must be assumed to have capacity unless it is established that he lacks capacity

s 1(3) A person is not to be treated as unable to make a decision unless all practicable steps to help him to do so have been taken without success

s 1(4) A person is not treated as unable to make a decision merely because he makes an unwise decision

s 1(5) An act done or decision made under this Act for or on behalf of a person who lacks capacity must be done, or made, in his best interests

s 1(6) Before the act is done, or the decision is made, regard must be had to whether the purpose for which it is needed can be as effectively achieved in a way that is less restrictive of the person's rights and freedom of action.

The Act has great importance for patients and their decision making and aims to empower people who lack 'capacity' to remain at the centre of the decision-making process and to safeguard them and the professionals who work with them. It makes it clear who can take decisions, in which situations, and how they should go about this. The Act also enables people to plan ahead for a time when they may lose capacity (NMC, 2007).

Further, the Act aims to ensure that people who lack 'capacity' are not abused, and it introduces a new criminal offence of neglect that can be the subject of a charge against anyone who has mistreated or wilfully neglected a person who lacks 'capacity'.

The Act is underpinned by a set of five key principles:

1. Presumption of capacity, where every adult has the right to make their own decisions and must be assumed to have capacity to do so unless it is proved otherwise.

2. The right for individuals to be supported to make their own decisions and to be given all appropriate help before anyone concludes that they cannot make their own decisions.

3. That individuals must retain the right to make decisions that may seem to others unwise or eccentric.

4. Best interests, where anything done for or on behalf of those without capacity must be in their best interests.

5. Least restrictive intervention, where anything done for or on behalf of those without capacity should be the least restrictive of their basic rights and freedoms. This links with the Human Rights Act 1998.

The Act deals with the issue of capacity and how this is to be assessed by carers and health care professionals. For health care professionals this assessment is essential when obtaining consent and is an important means of protecting oneself and the patient. Every adult therefore must be presumed to have the capacity to consent for treatment unless they are unable to take in or retain information provided about their treatment or care; unable to understand the information provided; or unable to weigh up the information as part of the decision-making process. Anyone can make the assessment and they must have 'reasonable belief' that the person is lacking capacity (NMC, 2007).

The Act addresses two situations where a designated decision-maker can act on behalf of someone who lacks capacity:

1. Lasting powers of attorney, which allows a person to appoint an attorney to act on their behalf if they should lose capacity in the future to make decisions about their health and welfare.

2. Court-appointed deputies who are able to make decisions on their behalf in regard to welfare, health care and financial matters, but this excludes refusal of consent to life-sustaining treatment. Deputies are appointed only if the Court cannot make a one-off decision to resolve the issues.

Establishing consent

Professional responsibility requires nurses to make the care of people their *first* concern and to ensure they gain consent before they begin treatment or care. This means that the process of establishing consent is rigorous, transparent, and demonstrates a clear level of professional accountability and an accurate record of all discussions and decisions relating to obtaining consent.

Informed consent is by definition consent given by the patient after a full and comprehensive explanation of the procedure is given. Consent should be sought by the practitioner who will carry out the procedure or someone who is capable of carrying out the procedure. For consent to be valid, a patient must be competent to make the necessary decision, be provided with sufficient information and act voluntarily.

Anything that is done to a patient must be carried out with the patient's consent in the first instance wherever possible. In health care, the information given must always be the first consideration of the health care professional, that they are indeed knowledgeable and able to provide sufficient information and that they are obtaining consent for a procedure that they themselves are carrying out.

> The rule of thumb for nurses is simple – the more complex the procedure the less likely that you would be obtaining consent, certainly on your own.

Valid consent must be given by a competent person (who may be a person lawfully appointed on behalf of the person) and must be given voluntarily. Another person cannot give consent for an adult who has the capacity to consent.

However, consent is something that we take for granted and that we acknowledge and accept in silence – for example, the patient familiar with the ward and its routines, who rolls up their sleeve or holds out their arm for their blood pressure to be taken. Contrast this with the patient who has never been in hospital or with the patient who is unfamiliar with such a routine assessment.

The process of consent requires health care professionals to provide the patient with as much information as is wished, in a language which can be understood, and then to give the patient the opportunity to reflect on this information and ask questions. This is vital where decision making results in accepting or refusing treatment. The NMC (2008a) reiterates the Mental Capacity Act: if the patient is unable to take in or retain, understand and weigh up the information as part of the decision-making process then they may not have the capacity to consent.

Establishing consent is not a one-off event but rather a process, and the complexity of this process reflects that of the procedure for which consent is being sought. When a person is told about proposed treatment and care, it is important that the information is given in a sensitive and understandable way and that sufficient time and opportunity are provided to consider the information and to ask questions if they wish to. Nurses and midwives should not assume that the person in their care has sufficient knowledge, even about basic treatment, for them to make a choice (NMC, 2008a).

The assessment of whether an adult lacks the capacity to consent is primarily down to the clinician providing the treatment or care, but nurses and midwives have a responsibility to participate in discussions about this assessment. Nurses and midwives have overriding professional responsibilities with regard to obtaining consent, which reflect professional standards of care.

Consent may be implied, oral or written. Verbal and written consent should always be obtained before any procedure is undertaken. The patient has the right to refuse consent to the presence of individuals from any discipline if they are considered to be non-essential to the procedure. Non-essential personnel may include medical and nursing students, paramedics in training as well as representatives of the medical devices industry. Failure to obtain informed consent from the patient for any clinical procedure, including taking photographs, could result in a charge of trespass against the person.

A further provision of the Mental Capacity Act 2010 addresses advance decisions to refuse treatment, providing clear safeguards to confirm that people may make a decision in advance to refuse treatment if they should lose capacity in the future. It is made clear in the Act that an advance decision will have no application to any treatment which a doctor considers necessary to sustain life unless strict formalities have been complied with. These formalities are that the decision must be in writing, signed and witnessed. In addition, there must be an express statement that the decision stands 'even if life is at risk' (NMC, 2007).

Patients can choose not to have treatment and it is important that this is reflected in decision making, communication and documentation, particularly in medicines management. The patient's ability and willingness to accept treatment and medicines prescribed are integral to medicines management; however, approximately 25–50 per cent of patients fail to follow prescribed treatments (WHO, 2003).

Compliance to treatment relates to both action and behaviour where concordance suggests equality and negotiation in the treatment process between the health care professional and the patient (Lawson and Hennefer, 2010). Compliance suggests that there has been discussion and the consensual process has been engaged with the patient, addressing key elements of validity and information giving.

We have to accept however, that some patients do not want or may be unwilling to make decisions about their treatment.

This raises the ethical and moral dilemmas that health care practitioners are presented with in daily practice and indeed in medicines management. It emphasises the importance of good communication, teamwork and documentation. It also addresses the importance of how well we are informed and how effectively we can elicit this understanding from patients, whether they agree or not, refuse or accept. We may not agree with their decisions or the outcome, however it is essential that we demonstrate a professional role and advocate where necessary, show respect at all times, not judge, and consider what acting in the best interests really means to patients.

The Human Rights Act 1998

The Human Rights Act 1998 is wide-ranging and promises that the state will respect the rights and freedoms of individuals. Human rights are very much a part of everyday life – as citizens, professionals, patients and clients (McHale and Gallagher, 2004). Nurses need to be aware of the potential implications of the Act for their practice and care provision.

ACTIVITY 6.4

Access the Human Rights Act 1998 from the web link www.opsi.gov.uk.

The Act applies to children (a person under the age of 18) as well as to adults where some of the articles impact on nursing practice: nurses are encouraged to act as advocates for their patients/clients, to safeguard standards of care and to speak out where the patient/client may be at risk.

The Code (NMC, 2008a) requires registrants to bring any circumstances that may compromise patient/client care and safety to the attention of an appropriate authority. This imposes a duty to abide by those articles of the Human Rights Act 1998 and provisions of the Mental Capacity Act 2010.

Key articles of the Human Rights Act 1998 which relate to health care are:

Article 2: Right to life

Article 3: Prohibition of torture

Article 8: Right to respect for private and family life

Article 9: Freedom of thought, conscience and religion.

Article 2 of the Human Rights Act reinforces our professional obligation and has clear implications for decisions regarding withholding and/or withdrawing of life-preserving or life-saving treatment. It must be clear, though, that there will always be challenges with regard to non-resuscitation orders and demands for more aggressive treatments for people with serious illness. Article 3 of the Act states no one shall be subject to torture or inhumane degrading treatment or punishment. Inhumane treatment is deemed to be any treatment that causes intense physical and mental suffering. Article 8 of the Act recognises an individual's right to private and family life subject to specific qualifications. The right to respect for private life is to be balanced against Article 10, the right to freedom of expression.

Confidentiality of personal patient information is protected by the Human Rights Act 1998 and the Data Protection Act 1995. All health care professionals and every employee of the NHS is expected to respect the duty of confidentiality, largely as a result of contracts of employment. However, nurses also have a professional duty of care to protect, and unauthorised breach of confidentiality of personal patient information could result in fitness-to-practise proceedings by the NMC.

The Data Protection Act 1998

Health care professionals should be aware of provisions for respecting patient confidentiality and data protection.

 ACTIVITY 6.5

Access the Data Protection Act 1998 from the web link www.opsi.gov.uk.

Consent to disclose patient information must be obtained and protection of patient information must be observed. The Data Protection Act 1998 is a fundamental statutory instrument that sets out those principles with which users of personal information must comply. The legislation also gives individuals the right to gain access to information held about them and provides for a supervisory authority to oversee and enforce the law. This applies to certain manual records (if they form part of a relevant filing system) as well as computerised records, personal and individual files, and most health records (Dimond, 2005). In relation to medicines management, patients need to be aware of and consent to patient information being shared among health care professionals. It is important that patients understand that sharing this information facilitates good clinical decision making about their treatment and care. However, it must be shared with the patient's consent.

The main provisions of the Data Protection Act 1998 are:

Part 1. Preliminary – Basic provisions and principles of the Act in its application.

Part 2. Rights of data subjects and others – Rights of access and prevention from misuse.

Part 3. Notification to the data controllers – Duty, power and functions of Commissioner.

Part 4. Exemptions – In regard to available information to the public, i.e. national security and disclosure required by law.

Part 5. Enforcement

Part 6. Miscellaneous and general – Listed schedules of the Act.

Health and safety

A final consideration in medicines management that has been underlying throughout this book is health and safety and management of risk, to us and to patients.

ACTIVITY 6.6

How is health and safety legislation reflected in your workplace?

....

....

....

....

....

....

Infection control and risk is a key area in health care that has been scrutinised and largely influenced by research. The NHS is making every effort to implement safe practice and reduce the risk of infection, introducing controls which have been predominantly influenced by research and guidelines that address asepsis and safe techniques in clinical practice. Adopting a 'non-touch' technique is a key strategy for all NHS trusts, particularly in medicine administration (Pratt et al., 2007) and routine clinical practice.

ACTIVITY 6.7

Access the *Epic 2: National Evidence-Based Guidelines for Preventing Healthcare-Associated Infections in NHS Hospitals in England* using the web link http://www.epic.tvu.ac.uk/PDFfiles/epic2/ epic2-final.pdf/_blank.

Hand-washing campaigns advocate good practice for *all* health care professionals, and seek to actively engage practitioners to promote and implement practices that will reduce infection and associated risks to patients.

Often, in practice, practitioners are faced with challenges, particularly in promoting safe practice and following such guidelines and protocols that are evidence and research based. It is essential that nurses feel they can challenge poor practice and advocate patient safety. The first step is having knowledge and the rationale for our actions and to be role models of good practice.

At times this may be difficult, and it is important for practitioners to feel supported when faced with such challenges. All health care providers are engaging with government initiatives that target a safer NHS. Therefore it is everyone's responsibility to actively promote safe practice. When patients are admitted to hospital they expect to receive quality nursing care – they do not expect to be harmed (Elliott and Liu, 2010). Patient harm as a result of health care interventions, or lack of effective preventative measures, can cause patients to lose confidence in the ability of the NHS to safely care for them (Pratt, 2005). Patients have a right to clean and safe treatment wherever and whenever they are treated by the NHS (Department of Health, 2008). The National Patient Safety Agency reports that avoidable harm occurs in hospitals across the world, and that more than one in ten people admitted to hospital are harmed unintentionally by its care (NPSA, 2008).

Medicines management is everyone's business and it requires safe, skilful and knowledgeable practice. It is imperative that patient safety comes first and that safety is embedded in our practice.

Tips for safe practice in medicines management

- The patient must come first!
  - Check the patient's identity against the prescription chart - this medicine could potentially be for the wrong patient
  - Administering medication to the wrong patient is a common error
  - Patient 'misidentification' is an identified source of error
- Know your patient!
  - The patient, their condition and the treatment should be appropriate and indicated for that patient
  - If the patient does not have an infection, ask yourself why have they been prescribed an antibiotic? Does the drug make sense for this patient?
- Protect your patient!
  - Hands must be washed
  - Adopt an aseptic non-touch technique
  - Wear non-sterile gloves when indicated and appropriate
- Keep what you have cleaned, clean!
  - Once the skin has been cleansed it should not be re-palpated
  - Allow time for the skin or equipment to dry naturally
- Understand what you are doing and why
  - Knowledge and skills are essential
  - If you are uncertain, it is your responsibility to seek advice from a reliable source or experienced practitioner
  - Follow organisation policies and recommended guidelines. Not knowing is not an excuse!
- Professional responsibility
  - It is your duty not to harm your patient
  - You must be proactive to ensure patient safety first.

STOP

THINK

QUESTION?

Chapter summary

Medicines management relies on health care professionals to have sound knowledge, skill and expertise and to use this as armour to protect patients and themselves. It is essential that nurses are confident in their clinical decision making and communication skills, which are fundamental to safe medicines management and patient care. Decisions need to be made in the patients' best interests, with the patients' consent wherever possible and in agreement with the carers, patients' families and the health care team.

Assessing patients' capacity to make decisions for themselves is essential, and a requirement wherever capacity is brought into question. The statutory instrument that provides guidance on assessment and clarifies capacity is the Mental Capacity Act 2010, and this should be read conjunction with the NMC Code (2008a) and the Human Rights Act 1998, which aim to protect the rights and freedoms of individuals and ensure that safe consensual decision making is happening in practice. This includes protecting the patient and their information and understanding the importance of confidentiality. Not all patients will want treatment, and it is their right to refuse - we need to be cautious and respectful of a patient's decisions and ensure that we have sought advice wherever and whenever we are uncertain in our practice and decision making. A key to good decisions is having insight, to ask, to question and to understand.

'Nurses armoured with knowledge' is the first step to safe practice and essential when clinical decision making is needed.

The NMC (2008a) indicates that nurses must justify their actions and their omissions. This requires an understanding of what it is we do and why. A significant catalyst to our actions comes from the rationale for what we do. This is highly influenced by evidence and indeed research that purposes to support our decision making and provide those reasons that help in our understanding for the decisions we make.

So what have you learned?

Let's do a quick check. Write down your answers to the following questions or simply tick whether the statement is true or false.

1. The Mental Capacity Act aims to protect vulnerable patients.

   True ☐   False ☐

2. List the three types of consent.

   ....

   ....

   ....

3. What makes consent valid?

   ....

   ....

4. Give an example of evidence-based practice in medicines management.

   ....

   ....

   ....

5. List three reliable sources to support practice.

   ....

   ....

   ....

References and key texts

Department of Health (2008) *Clean, Safe Care: Reducing Infections and Saving Lives*. London: The Stationery Office.

Dimond, B. (ed.) (2005) *Legal Aspects of Nursing*, 4th edn. Harlow: Pearson.

Elliott, M. and Liu, Y. (2010) 'The nine rights of medication administration: an overview'. *British Journal of Nursing* 19 (5): 300-5.

Elsaleh, H., Joseph, D., Grieu, F., Zeps, N., Spry, N. and Iacopetta, B. (2001) 'A spoonful of sugar - improving medicines management in hospitals: summary'. *British Journal of Surgery* 130: 17-20. Available at www.bmj.com/content/324/7343/931.full.pdf.

Lawson, E. and Hennefer, D.L. (2010) *Medicine Management*. Exeter: Learning Matters.

McHale, J. and Gallagher, A. (2004) *Nursing and the Human Rights*. London: Butterworth Heinemann.

National Prescribing Centre (2007) *A Competency Framework for Shared Decision-Making with Patients: Achieving Concordance for Taking Medicines*. Keele: NPC Plus.

NMC (Nursing and Midwifery Council) (2007) *Mental Capacity Act Summary*. London: NMC.

NMC (Nursing and Midwifery Council) (2008a) *The Code: Standards of Conduct, Performance and Ethics for Nurses and Midwives*. London: NMC.

NMC (Nursing and Midwifery Council) (2008b) *Standards for Medicines Management*. London: NMC.

NPSA (National Patient Safety Agency) (2008) *Reducing Dosing Errors with Opioid Medicines*. RRROS. Available at www.npsa.nhs.uk.

Pratt, R.J. (2005) Preventing Healthcare-associated Infections: An Essential Component of Patient Safety. Available at http://www.saferhealthcare.org.uk/HI/InfectionControl/WhatWeKnow.

Pratt, R.J., Pellowe, C.M., Wilson, J.A. et al. (2007) *Epic 2: National Evidence-Based Guidelines for Preventing Healthcare-Associated Infections in NHS Hospitals in England*. Available at *Journal of Hospital Infection* (Suppl.) 65 S: s1-s64.

WHO (World Health Organization) (2003) *Adherence to Long-Term Therapies: Evidence for Action*. Geneva: WHO: Available at http://www.who.int/publications/2003/9241545992.pdf.

Additional reading

Department of Health (2001a) *National Service Framework for Older People*. London: The Stationery Office.

Department of Health (2001b) *Medicines and Older People: Implementing Medicines-Related Aspects of the NSF for Older People*. London: The Stationery Office.

Dougherty, L. and Lister, S. (2008) *Royal Marsden Hospital Manual of Clinical Nursing Procedures*. Oxford: Wiley Blackwell.

Hewitt-Taylor, J. (2002) 'Evidence-based practice'. *Nursing Standard* 17: 47–52.

Hughes, S.L., Whittlesea, C. and Luscombe, D. (2002) 'Patient's knowledge and perceptions of the side-effects of OTC medication'. *Journal of Clinical Pharmacology and Therapeutics* 27: 243–8.

NHSIA (National Health Service Information Authority) (2002) *Share with Care: People's Views on Consent and Confidentiality of Patient Information*. NHSIA: London.

NMC (Nursing and Midwifery Council) (2010) *Record Keeping: Guidelines for Nurses and Midwives*. London: NMC.

NPSA (National Patient Safety Agency) (2004) *Seven Steps to Patient Safety: An Overview Guide for NHS Staff*. Available at http://www.npsa.co.uk/patientsafety/improvingpatientsafety/7steps/.

NPSA (National Patient Safety Agency) (2007) *Safety in Doses: Improving the Use of Medicines in the NHS*. Available at http://npsa.uk/patientsafety/medication-zone/reviews-of-medication-incidents/.

Royal College of Nursing (2008) *Nursing Our Future: An RCN Study into the Challenges Facing Today's Nursing Students in the UK*. London: RCN.

Walters, T.P. (2009) 'The Mental Capacity Act – a balance between protection and liberty'. *British Journal of Nursing* 18 (9): 555–8.

Welsh, S. and Deahl, M. (2002) 'Covert medication: ever ethically justifiable?' *Psychiatric Bulletin* 26: 123–6.

Wright, D. (2002) 'Swallowing difficulties protocol: medication administration'. *Nursing Standard* 17 (14/15): 43–5.

Websites

http://www.cqc.org.uk

http://www.dh.gov.uk

http://www.npsa.uk

http://www.opsi.gov.uk

http://www.saferhealthcare.org.uk

http://www.who.int

Answers to chapter questions

Chapter 1

Your starting point

1. Trustworthy; non-discriminatory; kind; considerate; helpful; respectful; good listener; competent; knowledgeable; professional; skilled; cooperative; fair; impartial.
2. Acting in a way that adheres to NMC standards of care and the Code.
3. Responsible can be defined as having a legal or moral obligation to take care of something or to carry out a duty.
4. Accountable can be defined as being responsible for something or to someone.
5. Yes
6. Unable to administer medicines without direct supervision as a student nurse.
7. Safe; competent; high standard of care; not to harm; advocate for; engage with and treat with respect and as a fellow human being.
8. Yes

So what have you learned?

1. True   2. True   3. False   4. True   5. True

Chapter 2

Your starting point

1. Working collectively and effectively to produce shared patient outcomes and goals.
2. Essential standards of care (NMC Code, 2008).
3. Lack of communication; not working together; unprofessional behaviour; lack of priority for the patient and their care.
4. Engage with members of the IPT and the patient(s); plan and deliver patient-focused care; work together with the same goals and patient outcomes.

5. Doctors; pharmacists; nurses; physiotherapists; occupational therapists; nutritionists; anaesthetists; phlebotomists; speech therapists, specialist nurses such as the pain team.
6. Work collaboratively within the IPT to promote health, provide treatment and care, and to manage patients.
7. Yes. Patient safety; promotion of health; management of patients; treatment and interventions; planning and delivering care; monitoring and evaluating the patient and their care.

So what have you learned?
1. Doctors; nurses; physiotherapists; occupational therapists; pharmacists; anaesthetists; specialist teams such as pain team; diabetic nurse specialists; nutritionists.
2. True
3. Communication; collaboration; working together with same goals for patient care.
4. True
5. Safety of patient care; recognise limits on what you can and cannot do.

Chapter 3

Your starting point
1. Awareness of unsafe practice, risk, processes of safe practice, policy and procedures to guide safe practice.
2. Work within limitations; follow policy and procedures and practice guidelines; seek support from experienced members of the IPT.
3. The Five Rights in medicine administration.
4. Yes
5. Patient identity.
6. Legislation - Medicines Act 1968, Misuse of Drugs Act 1971.
7. Medicines Act 1968.

So what have you learned?
1. True
2. Identify the correct patient; the correct prescription; the correct drug.
3. C
4. PO = sold by pharmacists; POM = need a prescription, authorised by a prescriber.
5. MHRA

Chapter 4

Your starting point

1. Error = mistake; being wrong in conduct or judgement.
   Mistake = same as an error.
2. Yes - same.
3. Wrong patient; wrong drug; wrong dose; wrong route; wrong time.
4. Check patient identity against the prescription chart and patient identity band; know and understand the drug prescribed for that patient at that time; select the correct drug.

So what have you learned?

1. True
2. Right patient, Right drug, Right dose, Right route, Right time.
3. 0-8 and 70-100 age groups.
4. *Standards for Medicines Management* (NMC, 2008) and *Guidelines for the Administration of Medicines* (NMC, 2004).
5. BNF
6. Half a tablet.

Chapter 5

Your starting point

1. A-C   B-A   C-B
2. Liver
3. The study of drugs and how they affect the host tissue or fight disease.
4. A-C   B-B   C-A
5. Kidney, lungs, faecal excretion, skin.
6. Fridge; patient's bedside locker; CD cupboard; medicine storage room on the ward and drug cupboards; medication trolley; arrest trolley.
7. Oramorph; MST; Sevredol; Morcap.
8. No

So what have you learned?

1. True
2. True
3. Absorption; Distribution; Metabolism; Excretion.
4. Morphine

5. Naloxone
6. A-C   B-A   C-B
7. Intravenous route.
8. Bruising; infection; phlebitis; infiltration; extravasation.

Chapter 6

Your starting point

1. Drug Policy; NMC; RCN; BNF.
2. Did not check the patient identity; wrong prescription for the patient.
3. Language; information given at a pace the patient can understand; risks and benefits explained clearly; patient able to retain the information and have the opportunity to ask questions; the patient can agree to the treatment or refuse.
4. No
5. Yes

So what have you learned?

1. True
2. Verbal; implied; written.
3. The patient can agree to treatment or refuse.
4. Epic 2 guidelines; RCN guidelines; NMC Code.
5. NMC Code; trust policies and procedures for medicines management; BNF.

Glossary

Absorption The point of drug interaction whereby the drug is transferred from the site of administration to the general circulation.

Accountable Responsible for something or to someone.

Active transport The movement of a substance against its concentration energy.

Adverse effect Unknown effects such as anaphylaxis as a result of drug interaction in the body.

Affinity Drug-binding ability.

Agonist Stimulates the receptor and produces an effect similar to that of naturally occurring stimuli. Agonists may be *full*, *partial* or *inverse*.

Air embolism Air entering into the vascular system.

Anaphylaxis Exaggerated allergic response that can be life threatening.

Antagonist Blocks the action of the agonist.

Autonomy Respecting the decision-making capacities of autonomous persons.

Beneficence Balancing of benefits.

Bioavailability The ability of a drug to be absorbed and reach the site of action.

Boundaries Barriers or limitations to what one can do within one's role.

Buccal Drug route when a drug is placed into the pouch of the cheek.

Capacity One's ability to understand, comprehend and have the faculties to make a decision for oneself and about oneself.

Cardiac arrhythmia Abnormal heart rate or rhythm.

Consent Process of giving information that clearly explains the risks and benefits of the proposed treatment, in a way in which someone can understand, ask questions, and refuse or accept.

Creatinine clearance rate Identifies the volume of blood plasma that is cleared of creatinine per unit time.

Diffusion The movement of molecules or particles across a cell membrane.

Distribution Where the drug goes in the body in order to enter systemic circulation.

Efficacy The ability of the drug to affect the receptor and cause a response after binding.

Elimination Removal of a drug from the body when the drug action terminates.

Evidence-based Research and evidence that supports and shapes clinical practice.

Extravasation Vesicant fluid leakage into tissue outside of a vein.

Haemorrhage Bleeding or abnormal blood flow.

Half-life The amount of time the body takes to eliminate a drug.

Infection Contamination caused by microbes.

Infiltration Fluid leakage into tissues outside of a vein.

Inhalation A drug route, taken in through nose or mouth when breathing.

Intramuscular A drug route, injected into muscle tissue.

Intravenous A drug route direct into systemic circulation.

Justice Distributing benefits, risks and costs fairly.

Metabolism Breaking down or detoxifying drugs into a usable or soluble form by liver enzymes.

Negligence Any act of carelessness, lack of regard or lack of insight which can lead to patient harm.

Nomenclature The naming of drugs.

Non-maleficence Avoiding the causation of harm to the patient.

Non-vesicant Medicines or fluids that are not irritable to the vein such as 0.9% sodium chloride.

Pharmacodynamics The study of how drugs act and of what the drug does to the body.

Pharmacokinetics The study of what the body does to the drug and the effects of the body on drug delivery to its site of action.

Pharmacology The study of how drugs affect the function of host tissues or combat infectious organisms.

Phlebitis Inflammation of the vein.

Pneumothorax Collection of air or gas in the pleural cavity of the chest between the lung and the chest wall.

Professional Proficiently skilled, trained and practised.

Rectal In medicine administration, drugs in the form of a suppository can be inserted into the rectum where the drug is readily absorbed through the thin vascular wall of the rectal mucosa.

Responsible A legal or moral obligation to take care of something or to carry out a duty.

Side effect Known effects of the drug such as gastrointestinal upset, that the drug may cause as a result of its action and therapeutic efficacy.

Solubility The ability of compounds to dissolve, where fat or lipids are generally not soluble in water.

Subcutaneous A drug route injection used for a slow, sustained absorption of medication (0.5 to 2 ml), injected into the subcutaneous tissue.

Sublingual A drug route under the tongue.

Teamwork In relation to medicines management, two or more health care professionals sharing a common goal, with a balanced contribution of expertise, working collaboratively in mutual support.

Thrombosis The formation of a blood clot inside a blood vessel that can obstruct blood flow through the circulatory system.

Topical In medicine administration, a topical medication is applied to body surfaces such as the skin or mucous membranes such as the vagina, anus, throat, eyes and ears which are collectively 'topical' in their route.

Vascular access device A catheter device inserted into a vein.

Vesicant Medicines or fluids that can be irritating to the vein when administered, for example potassium chloride, 5 per cent sodium bicarbonate, antibiotics, cytotoxics.

Index

Figures and tables are in italics; terms defined in the Glossary are in bold

Index

Printed and bound by CPI Group (UK) Ltd, Croydon, CR0 4YY

23/10/2024

01778241-0002